Advancing Healthcare Through Data-Driven Innovations

Advancing Healthcare Through Data-Driven Innovations

Editors

Gunjan
Department of Computer Science and Engineering
National Institute of Technology, Delhi, India

Aditya Gupta
Department of Electrical and Instrumentation Engineering
Thapar Institute of Engineering and Technology, Patiala, India

Vibha Jain
Department of Computer Science and Engineering
Thapar Institute of Engineering and Technology Patiala, India

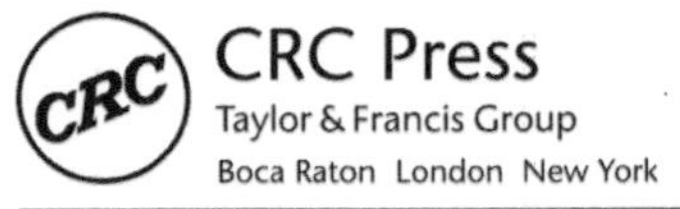

CRC Press
Taylor & Francis Group
Boca Raton London New York

CRC Press is an imprint of the
Taylor & Francis Group, an **informa** business

A SCIENCE PUBLISHERS BOOK

First edition published 2025
by CRC Press
2385 NW Executive Center Drive, Suite 320, Boca Raton FL 33431

and by CRC Press
4 Park Square, Milton Park, Abingdon, Oxon, OX14 4RN

© 2025 Gunjan, Aditya Gupta and Vibha Jain

CRC Press is an imprint of Taylor & Francis Group, LLC

Library of Congress Cataloging-in-Publication Data (applied for)

ISBN: 978-1-032-73717-1 (hbk)
ISBN: 978-1-032-75726-1 (pbk)
ISBN: 978-1-003-47539-2 (ebk)

DOI: 10.1201/9781003475392

Typeset in Times New Roman
by Prime Publishing Services

Preface

Welcome to "Advances in Healthcare Through Data-Driven Innovations." In this book, we embark on an illuminating journey into the transformative realm where cutting-edge technologies intersect with the timeless pursuit of better health and wellness. The landscape of healthcare is rapidly evolving, propelled by the relentless march of innovation and the transformative power of data-driven technologies such as blockchain, artificial intelligence (AI), big data analytics, and machine learning.

Data-driven solutions have become important in the constantly evolving healthcare industry. In the current state of medicine, where technology and patient care are closely connected, it is crucial to have a thorough understanding of data-driven methods.

"Advancing Healthcare Through Data-Driven Innovations" investigates the convergence between healthcare and technological advances, specifically focusing on how data analytics, artificial intelligence, and machine learning are transforming the industry as a whole. The potential of these developments is endless, ranging from improved diagnostic accuracy to improving treatment outcomes.

This book provides guidance for healthcare practitioners, academics, policymakers, and technologists in understanding and managing the intricate landscape of data-driven healthcare. By following a series of enlightening chapters written by professionals in their various domains, readers will acquire a more profound comprehension of the revolutionary influence of data and its consequences for the future of medicine.

Every chapter presents a distinct viewpoint, examining a wide range of uses from predictive analytics in tailored medicine to the ethical concerns related to data privacy and security. This book provides readers with the required information and techniques to effectively utilize data-driven innovations in healthcare by analyzing real-world case studies and the latest research.

What's in the Book?

Chapter 1 entitled *"Big Data's Impact on Healthcare Transformation"* emphasizes the role of big data in accelerating medical research. It also highlights personalized medicine fuelled by patient-centric data, predictive analytics shaping proactive treatments, and the optimization of hospital operations through data-driven insights. This chapter will serve as a starting point for beginners to learn the impact and significance of big data in the healthcare industry irrespective of their domains.

Chapter 2 entitled *"Healthcare with COVID-19: Artificial Intelligence and Machine Learning Techniques"* explores medical datasets for dementia detection using machine learning and highlights the growing interdisciplinary applications of machine learning. Its primary objective is to demonstrate the potential of machine learning in healthcare and other sectors, showcasing recent advancements and future possibilities.

Chapter 3 entitled *"Predictive analytics tools and techniques for Disease prevention and early detection in the healthcare sector"* discusses the benefits, challenges, and best practices of prediction algorithms in healthcare, highlighting their role in enhancing prevention and early detection efforts and delving into the capabilities of predictive analytics tools and methods.

Chapter 4 entitled *"Machine learning-based analysis for detection of pancreatic adenocarcinoma using urinary biomarkers"* investigates the use of urinary biomarkers for early detection of pancreatic cancer, a challenging disease often diagnosed in advanced stages. Various ensemble methods like bagging and AdaBoost are also explored to improve predictive accuracy, offering valuable insights for non-invasive pancreatic cancer diagnosis.

Chapter 5 entitled *"Gland Segmentation in Colon Histology Images Using Deep Learning Method"* introduces the U-Net model, a deep-learning technique, for segmenting glandular structures in colon histological images. Leveraging the U-Net architecture, known for its efficacy in medical image analysis, and the Warwick-QU dataset, expertly annotated with hematoxylin and eosin staining, the study accurately identifies malignant tissues in colon histology images.

Chapter 6 entitled *"Comparative Analysis for Detecting Cancer in Various Organs using Cellular Automata based Segmentation Technique"* utilizes cellular automata and machine learning techniques to detect cancer in various organs, including the brain, breast, and skin. By analyzing medical images and identifying aberrant cell growth regions, automated cancer detection is achieved. Comparative analysis with original image sets highlights the effectiveness of the approach in early and accurate cancer detection, emphasizing its potential to save lives.

Chapter 7 entitled *"Convolutional Neural Networks and Transfer Learning for Medical Image Analysis: A Comprehensive Review"* provides a comprehensive examination of CNNs and Transfer Learning (TL) techniques in medical imaging, highlighting their contributions to disease detection and treatment planning. It underscores the effectiveness of CNNs in medical image classification and advocates for further research to enhance CNN and TL methods in medical imaging, outlining potential future research directions.

Chapter 8 entitled *"Multi-objective optimization enabled improved feature selection"* comprehensively analyzes the multi-objective feature selection problem and evaluates various strategies to address it. The review serves as a comprehensive repository of strategies and methodologies for multi-objective feature selection, while also identifying ongoing challenges and suggesting areas for future research.

Chapter 9 entitled *"IoT-Blockchain in Remote Pregnancy Care Coordination"* explores the integration of Internet of Things (IoT) and blockchain technologies in Remote Pregnancy Monitoring (RPM) to improve healthcare for expectant mothers. It presents a systematic review of current RPM applications and proposes a novel framework tailored to remote pregnancy care.

Chapter 10 entitled *"Strengthening Healthcare Data Security and Privacy"* emphasizes the importance of blockchain in securing healthcare systems and outlines a roadmap for its implementation and future impact.

Chapter 11 entitled *"The Future of Healthcare: Data-Driven Trends and Innovation"* examines the future of medical care, emphasizing the transformative potential of innovations in technology. It also explores how IoT devices and sensors can monitor vital signs, track conditions, and gather health data, as well as the role of IoT in healthcare.

Contents

List of Contributors

Aakansha Gupta
Delhi Technological University, New Delhi, India.

Aarushi Gupta
Rajmata Vijaya Raje Scindia Medical College, Bhilwara.

Aaryan Gupta
Manipal University Jaipur, Jaipur.

Adarsh Kumar Arya
Department of Chemical Engineering, Harcourt Butler Technical University, Kanpur, India.

Aditi Sharma
Department of Artificial Intelligence, School of Computer Science & Engineering, Manipal University, Jaipur, India.

Aleena Swetapadma
School of Computer Engineering, KIIT Deemed to be University, Bhubaneswar, India.

Ashish Kapoor
Department of Chemical Engineering, Harcourt Butler Technical University, Kanpur, India.

Biswajit Sahoo
School of Computer Engineering, KIIT Deemed to be University, Bhubaneswar, India.

Devanshi Srivastava
Department of Chemical Engineering, Harcourt Butler Technical University, Kanpur, India.

Hemlata Parmar
Department of Artificial Intelligence, School of Computer Science & Engineering, Manipal University, Jaipur, India.

Jayesh Gangrade
Department of Artificial Intelligence, School of Computer Science & Engineering, Manipal University, Jaipur, India.

M. Mohan
Associate Professor, Computer Science Engineering, SRM University, Delhi NCR, India.

Mahruf Islam Prottoy
   Software Engineer, Millennium Solutions, Dhaka, Bangladesh.
Manjulata Badi
   Assistant Professor, EEE Department, Alliance University, Bangalore, India
Md. Samin Morshed
   Graduate Student, University of Arkansas at Little Rock, Arkansas, U.S.A.
Mohammad Mobarak Hossain
   PhD Fellow, DUET, Gazipur, Bangladesh.
Mohammod Abul Kashem
   Professor, Department of Computer Science and Engineering, DUET, Gazipur, Bangladesh.
Muhammad Usama Islam
   Lecturer, Asian University of Bangladesh, Bangladesh.
Nazma B. J. Naskar
   JIS University, WB, India.
Poojasri Inagala
   Department of Artificial Intelligence, School of Computer Science & Engineering, Manipal University, Jaipur, India.
Prakash Kuppuswamy
   Associate Professor, Computer Science Engineering, SRM University, Delhi NCR, India.
Prakhar Pipersania
   KIIT University, Odisha, India.
Rahul Katarya
   Delhi Technological University, New Delhi, India.
Rohit Singh
   Manipal University, Jaipur, India.
Rupashri Barik
   JIS College of Engineering, Kalyani, WB, India.
Samarpan Chandra
   KIIT University, Odisha, India.
Samudraneel Banerjee
   KIIT University, Odisha, India.
Satya Subham Nayak
   School of Computer Engineering, KIIT Deemed to be University, Bhubaneswar, India.
Sayed QY Al Khalidi
   Professor, Department of Information Technology, King Khalid University, Abha, KSA.
Shalini Basak
   KIIT University, Odisha, India.
Shashwat Jha
   KIIT University, Odisha, India.

Shreya
Department of Chemical Engineering, Harcourt Butler Technical University, Kanpur, India

Shroddha Ghosh
School of Computer Engineering, KIIT Deemed to be University, Bhubaneswar, India

Vibha Jain
Thapar Institute of Engineering and Technology Patiala, India.

Vijaya Varshini Prakash
PG Student, Palaniappa College of Arts & Science, Bharathiyar University, T.N., India.

Vinay Dubey
Delhi Technological University, New Delhi, India.

Wasswa Shafik
School of Digital Science, Universiti Brunei Darussalam, Gadong, BE1410, Brunei Darussalam, Dig Connectivity Research Laboratory (DCRLab), Kampala, Uganda.

1

Big Data's Impact on Healthcare Transformation

Aaryan Gupta[1]* and *Aarushi Gupta*[2]

Set off on a revolutionary adventure in healthcare propelled by the potent energy of big data. Discover the world of personalized medicine, where patient-centric data is used to build precise treatment methods as predictive analytics ushers in a proactive therapeutic era. See how big data is essential for streamlining patient flow, improving hospital operations, and allocating resources for better treatment. Investigate the cutting edge of medical research, solving genetic puzzles and accelerating clinical trials with never-before-seen efficiency. Big data is the watchful protector of public health, allowing for quick diagnosis, containment, and flexible policy development for community safety. This abstract extends an invitation to scholars, professionals, and amateurs to join the data symphony and investigate the technical wonders of big data for patient-centered healthcare, which will enhance patient outcomes, empower decision-makers, and improve the state of world health. Come along on our journey towards a day when big data completely changes the healthcare industry.

Introduction

Understanding Big Data

Patient care and medical practices have changed dramatically as a result of the introduction of Big Data Analytics (BDA) into the complex field of healthcare.

[1] Manipal University Jaipur, Jaipur
[2] Rajmata Vijaya Raje Scindia Medical College, Bhilwara
* Corresponding author: aaryangupta1200@gmail.com

This chapter does a thorough analysis, utilizing the corpus of prior research as well as the empirical results of independent study projects to present a story that goes beyond traditional healthcare paradigms (Johnson and Miller, 2021).

Setting the Big Data Paradigm in Context

All industries have been touched by the current flood of organized and unstructured data, including the healthcare industry. A paradigm shift in data management is evident in the contrast between structured data, which adheres to set patterns and utilizes known processing formats, and unstructured Big Data, which defies established techniques. Integrating many data sources has the potential to significantly increase value inside medical organizations (Ghaleb et al., 2022).

Meaning of Big Data Analytics in the Medical Field

The central idea of this revolutionary era, big data analytics, has the key to extracting information from massive and heterogeneous datasets. In the healthcare industry, big data takes on a life of its own as a constantly evolving collection of methods and instruments that facilitate the extraction of relevant data from the vast big data universe. It does more than just data processing. As data analytics becomes increasingly integrated into the healthcare industry, it has the potential to forecast future health trends, provide individualized care, and identify complex clusters and links within patient records (Davis and Carter, 2021).

Opportunities and Difficulties: A Worldwide Conversation

The challenges that Big Data Analytics presents for the healthcare sector are discussed in this chapter. Using patient-data correlations, analyzing unstructured clinical notes, and efficiently handling massive volumes of medical imaging data are just a few of the many difficulties. There are several opportunities available at the same time, such as enhancing clinical procedures, expediting public health activities, and offering personalized care (Liu and Li, 2022).

An Analytical Journey Up Next

This chapter, broken up into distinct sections, approaches analysis from a wide perspective, focusing on more than just one particular technology. It examines the evolution of doctor-patient interactions, changes in healthcare systems, shifts in the roles of medical personnel, and the importance of a patient-centric healthcare paradigm (Edison, 2023).

The Evolution of Big Data in Healthcare

Historical Perspective: Unveiling the Roots of Transformation

An amazing tale of development is big data's historical development in health-care. Historically, typewritten reports or handwritten notes were used to meticulously record medical information; the earliest case reports were created in Egypt in 1600 BC. Clinical case records, according to Stanley Reiser, "froze the episode of illness as a story," in which patients, doctors, and families all had a part to play (Shamshari and Najaf, 2021).

The creation of computer systems, which promoted the digitization of clinical evaluations and medical data, was a significant turning point. The National Academies of Sciences, Engineering, and Medicine coined the term "electronic health records" (EHRs) in 2003 to describe computerized medical data used to improve patient care. Transitioning from paper-based to EHRs has several advantages, such as improved access to patient histories, more effective care coordination, less errors, and superior treatment (Thomson and Anderson, 2021).

Current Trends: Navigating the Landscape of Possibilities

Big data in healthcare goes beyond EHRs, with applications, genomics, and mobile biometric sensors adding to the richness of data. Proposals such as "All of Us" promote individualized treatment by gathering a large amount of patient data. Large datasets are made available by biomedical technologies, improving medical treatment, procedures, and technology. The goals of clinical transformation and healthcare analytics include better treatment planning, lower costs, and fraud prevention through effective Clinical Decision Support (CDS) systems. As medical data continues to grow, data privacy concerns remain along with a need for creative methods of integration, analysis, and interpretation (Cooper and Ward, 2022).

Future Prospects: Paving the Way for Predictive Healthcare

The rising use of big data in healthcare depends on how analytics, health informatics, and bioinformatics are used to solve the problem of combining structured and unstructured data. Expanding genetic data is driving the integration of physiological data with "-omics" techniques to construct a full human body model. Even with the difficulties in combining various medical datasets, the path leads to a sophisticated predictive healthcare system. Predicting health concerns, getting insights into population health, and estimating future results based on available data are critical. These steps usher in a new era of proactive healthcare that includes biomarker discovery, early warning systems, and creative therapies (Wang and Wang, 2020).

Conclusions and Future Prospects: Bridging Innovation and Challenges

The explosion of biomedical and healthcare data from sensors, cellphones, and genomes calls for comprehension. A precise prediction framework is shaped by collaborative analysis of EHRs and Electronic Medical Records (EMRs) in an effort to save costs, fight fraud, and enhance CDS systems. Personal data management still presents challenges, but computer system integration for healthcare signal processing is becoming more common. Predictive systems are promised by big data analytics in healthcare, which is moving to specific fields. Standards and privacy remain challenges despite progress, necessitating cooperation for best usage in diagnosis and treatment (C´wiklicki et al., 2021).

Applications of Big Data in Healthcare

The integration of big data in healthcare is propelling a new wave of innovative applications that are revolutionizing medical research development, hospital administration, and patient care. In this section, the many applications of big data in healthcare are reviewed, with an emphasis on four key areas: patient care, hospital management, medical research, and public health monitoring.

Medical Attention

Personalized Medicine

The field of personalized medicine is one where the implications of big data for patient care are particularly apparent. Medical professionals may use extensive databases to tailor treatment based on each patient's unique genetic makeup, lifestyle decisions, and medical background. Over time, better patient outcomes result from minimizing adverse effects and increasing treatment efficacy at the same time (Carter and Reynolds, 2022).

The Use of Predictive Analytics in Healthcare

Predicting potential health issues and their effects requires big data-driven predictive analytics. By studying large databases, medical practitioners may find high-risk individuals, predict the onset of a disease, and take preventative measures. This proactive approach reduces the severity of illnesses and improves patients' overall well-being by facilitating early intervention (Azam, 2022).

Hospital Administration

Resource Allocation

Making the best use of the resources at hand is necessary for the finest hospital administration. Big data makes it easier to analyze historical patient data, which helps hospitals plan ahead for peak hours, staff patients effectively, and keep track of medical supplies. The efficient allocation of resources based on data ensures smooth hospital operations, particularly when managing varying demand (Weerasinghe et al., 2023).

Optimizing Patient Flow

Big data makes it easier to optimize patient flow in hospitals. Healthcare facilities may improve their processes by monitoring admission and discharge patterns, bed occupancy rates, and patient movement in real time. Reduced wait times improve patient happiness and increase the overall effectiveness of healthcare delivery (Korayim et al., 2024).

Research in Medicine

Genomic Research

Big data is changing the landscape of medical research, especially in the field of genomics. Researchers may find genetic predispositions to illnesses, possible therapeutic targets, and individualized therapy regimens by analyzing large genomic databases. Precision medicine has immense potential at the nexus of big data and genetics (Praveen et al., 2022).

Clinical Trial Optimization

Reorganizing trial processes and guaranteeing real-time observation. Through the examination of several parameters such as patient demographics and electronic health data, researchers may enhance the efficacy and efficiency of clinical trials, therefore expediting the release of new pharmaceuticals into the market (Secinaro et al., 2021).

Public Health Monitoring

Disease Tracking and Surveillance

Thanks to big data, public health workers now have the resources necessary to efficiently identify and track illnesses. Authorities can detect possible outbreaks, focus treatments, and halt the spread of infectious illnesses by using extensive statistics on population health, travel patterns, and environmental variables (Dipietro et al., 2023).

Health Policy Planning

Big data is essential in forming healthcare strategies since it takes into account variables including the prevalence of diseases, changes in the population, and patterns of healthcare use. This flexibility guarantees that programs may adjust to changing public needs. In conclusion, big data and healthcare have a symbiotic connection that influences patient care, hospital administration, medical research, and public health monitoring. As technology advances, this link will likely promote innovation, enhance patient outcomes, and influence the direction of the medical industry (Furstenau et al., 2023).

Challenges in Implementing Big Data in Healthcare

The integration of Big Data into the complex network of healthcare systems poses a number of challenges that require careful consideration and well-considered solutions. This section examines the many obstacles that obstruct Big Data's seamless incorporation into the healthcare sector.

Uncertainty in Big Data Analytics

The inherent unpredictability that comes with Big Data analytics in the healthcare industry is one of its main challenges. Clinical records, medical imaging, and patient-generated data are all included in the dynamic and diversified pool of healthcare data. These elements provide difficulties for traditional analytics techniques to address. To manage uncertainty and ensure the accuracy of the insights generated for clinical decision-making, sophisticated statistical models and algorithms that can handle the intricacies of healthcare data must be developed (Cruz, 2020).

Data Privacy and Security Concerns

Data security and privacy are becoming increasingly important since the amount of healthcare data is increasing at an exponential rate. Strict access controls, secure data storage practices, and encryption are all necessary to protect sensitive patient data. It's challenging to strike a balance between stringent security procedures and medical professionals' ability to access data; this calls for constant ingenuity and attention to detail (Rao et al., 2022).

Data Integration and Interoperability

Wearable technology and EHRs are two examples of the diverse healthcare data sources that provide a significant barrier to successful integration and interoperability. The challenge lies not just in gathering data from various sources but also in integrating divergent standards and data formats. To obtain complete insights across the treatment continuum, uniform data structures and interoperable solutions must be developed. Standardization efforts are crucial to breaking down data silos, enabling seamless data flow, and promoting collective decision-making (Hassan et al., 2021).

Need for Skilled Personnel

Depending on how knowledgeable the workforce is about advanced analytics and technology, healthcare organizations may reap the most benefits from Big Data. It is critically necessary for healthcare workers to upskill in order to effectively harness the potential of big data. The use of data-driven methodologies in healthcare will require a planned approach to workforce development, together with targeted training programs and educational initiatives.

Overcoming Blockchain Implementation Barriers

Although it has its own set of operational challenges, blockchain technology is being heralded as a workable way to enhance the security and integrity of medical data. its successful application in healthcare. This means addressing issues with scalability, legal frameworks, and industry acceptance (Tunc-Abubakar et al., 2023).

Ethical Considerations in Data Utilization

The increasing use of Big Data in healthcare decision-making raises moral concerns around the proper use of patient data. To balance using data for medical advancements with preserving patient autonomy and privacy, a clever approach is required. Establishing governance frameworks and moral standards is crucial to guiding the ethical use of big data in healthcare and fostering community and patient trust.

Integration with Existing Healthcare Infrastructure

A major obstacle confronting healthcare technology is the seamless incorporation of Big Data technologies into the existing framework. Healthcare businesses have challenges in implementing and utilizing Big Data technologies due to old systems, varied data formats, and varying degrees of digital maturity. Strategy and gradual implementation are necessary to ensure a smooth transition and prevent disruptions in the delivery of healthcare (Hammami et al., 2024).

Regulatory Compliance and Legal Frameworks

Successful use of big data technology requires negotiating the complex legal and regulatory environment in the healthcare industry. The US Health Insurance Portability and Accountability Act (HIPAA) is a prime example of how important it is to abide by data privacy laws. To balance innovation and regulatory compliance, policymakers, healthcare groups, and technology vendors need to continue cooperating.

Cost and Resource Allocation

Implementing and maintaining a Big Data infrastructure in healthcare requires significant financial investments. Purchasing state-of-the-art technology, hiring highly skilled personnel, and ensuring regular system updates come with hefty costs. Healthcare businesses must balance maximizing resource allocation with ensuring the long-term viability of Big Data efforts.

Change Management and Cultural Shift

Introducing Big Data technologies in healthcare often requires a cultural shift. Overcoming resistance to change and fostering a creative culture, effective change management, and stakeholder engagement are essential for successful integration. Beyond technological hurdles, collaboration among lawmakers, medical experts, IT specialists, and the workforce it is crucial to address challenges in healthcare.

Overcoming these obstacles is imperative to unlock big data's revolutionary potential for improving patient outcomes, accelerating healthcare delivery, and advancing medical research (Omoyiola, 2023).

Machine Learning-based Secured Analysis for Smart Healthcare

Here, we examine the critical field of medical record protection within the framework of the expansive Internet of Things (IoT). The fast growth of technology, particularly the usage of IoT in the healthcare business, has resulted in personalized and speedy access to healthcare services. However, increased technological integration also brings with it challenges related to security, privacy, and naturally sensitive health data.

On-line Healthcare Monitoring System with Enhanced Security Measures

Here, we introduce a state-of-the-art online healthcare monitoring system that collects and analyzes patient health data via a network of sensors and medical devices. Water-marking and signal enhancements are examples of contemporary security approaches used to reinforce the system's performance and security components. An extensive analysis of the challenges brought on by manipulated data transfer is carried out, emphasizing how important it is to maintain data integrity in healthcare data aggregation techniques (Chen et al., 2014).

Collaborative and Intelligent Security Model for IoT-based Healthcare Environments

This section offers a cooperative and intelligent security architecture to address the many security risks connected to a variety of IoT-enabled healthcare systems. The model incorporates several machine learning methods to safely classify patient data, emphasizing the latest developments in the field. It includes an in-depth analysis of incorrectly installed hardware and network setups, as well as the complexities of safeguarding medical data against fraudulent traffic (Arora et al., 2023).

Machine Learning Techniques for Big Data Analysis in Healthcare IoT

The convergence of big data and the Internet of Things (IoT) has ushered in a new age in healthcare by offering unparalleled opportunities for data-driven patient care and decision-making. Within this paradigm, machine learning (ML) emerges as a crucial enabler, providing advanced tools for drawing meaningful conclusions from vast and diverse datasets. In the framework of the Internet of Medical Devices, we examine certain machine learning techniques intended for large-scale data analytics in this section.

ML-based Recommendation Systems in Healthcare

Personalized Treatment Recommendations

Advances in machine learning have enabled personalized therapeutic recommendations, which have fundamentally transformed the healthcare sector. Through the analysis of large-scale datasets containing patient genetic and medical histories, machine learning algorithms can detect intricate patterns that might be used to enhance and personalize healthcare practices. Using compelling case studies, we examine how recommendation algorithms impact treatment plan optimization and improved patient outcomes (Brooks and Parker, 2021).

Drug Discovery and Prescription Optimization

Machine learning techniques have revolutionized prescription optimization and medication discovery processes. By sifting through massive databases, these computers identify potential drug candidates, predict interactions, and improve prescribing techniques This article examines the methods underpinning these applications, shedding light on how machine learning (ML) is improving medication development and prescription practices in medicine.

Predictive Analytics in Healthcare with Machine Learning

Predictive analytics is a vital component of big data applications and is essential to the Internet of medical things. This subject's primary focus is on the use of machine learning-based prediction systems to forecast patient outcomes, disease trends, and resource consumption (Thomson and Anderson, 2022).

Forecasting Disease Outbreaks

Machine learning algorithms are used to examine large-scale healthcare datasets in order to predict and minimize disease outbreaks. Real-world case studies demonstrate the impact of timely predictions on public health initiatives and their effectiveness. This study clarifies the potential synergies between machine learning and predictive analytics to enhance healthcare preparedness.

Patient Outcome Prediction

Predicting patient outcomes involves a comprehensive analysis of machine learning models that use a range of health variables. Proactive healthcare treatments can result from better prediction accuracy through the combination of real-time data from wearables and IoT devices. This section provides an overview of the revolutionary potential of advanced machine learning applications for predicting patient outcomes (Din et al., 2023).

Machine Learning for Data Aggregation in Healthcare IoT

Effective data aggregation is necessary to get meaningful insights from IoT data in the healthcare industry. In order to solve real-time processing and storage concerns, this section looks into ML-based techniques for data aggregation.

Real-time Data Compression Techniques

We study real-time data compression techniques for the Internet of Medical Things (IOMT) based on machine learning. Adaptive algorithms minimize data volume without losing critical information, maximizing system efficiency. This section explains the intricacies of these techniques and how they support dependable and scalable healthcare IoT systems.

Cluster-based Self-Organizing Data Aggregation

We conduct an exploration into the use of cluster-based self-organizing algorithms for the aggregation of medical data. Machine learning enhances the scalability and reliability of these approaches, facilitating the efficient accumulation of data in large-scale IoT installations. We draw attention to how ML might improve data aggregation processes for reliable IoT healthcare systems.

Conclusion

Healthcare is changing as a result of big data integration in patient care, hospital administration, medical research, and public health monitoring. This chapter examines the broad implications of big data, demonstrating how proactive healthcare using predictive analytics and exact therapy matching may revolutionize personalized medicine. Big data enhances operational efficiency in hospital administration by optimizing patient flow and resource allocation. Big data speeds up precision medicine and drug development in the medical field, especially in genomics and clinical trials. It transforms the monitoring of public health, supporting the tracking and control of diseases. The chapter highlights big data's creativity and prospects, imagining improved patient outcomes and well-informed decision-making. Future research and cooperation will be guided by recommendations that are in line with the five Vs of big data. The storyline presents big data as a transformative force in the healthcare industry, influencing a future where data drives ongoing innovation and better results.

References

Arora N., Singh A., Shahare V. and Datta G. 2023. Introduction to Big Data Analytics. In Towards the Integration of IoT, Cloud and Big Data: Services, Applications and Standards (pp. 1–18). Singapore: Springer Nature Singapore.

Azam B. 2022. Big Data's Evolution: From Storage to Cloud-Driven Insights. *International Journal of Computer Science and Technology*, 6(2), 106–20.

Brooks A. and Parker L. 2021. Bridging Bytes and Business: A Research Inquiry into Big Data's Strategic Significance. *European Journal of Computer Science and Information Technology*, 9(1), 71–78.

C´wiklicki M., Duplaga, M. and Klich, J. (Eds.). 2021. *The digital transformation of healthcare: Health* 4.0. Routledge.

Carter E. and Reynolds M. 2022. The interplay of data and algorithms: Big data influence on artificial intelligence. *EPH-International Journal of Mathematics and Statistics*, 8(2), 1–4.

Chen M., Mao S. and Liu Y. 2014. Big data: A survey. Mobile networks and applications, 19, 171–209.

Cooper L. and Ward G. 2022. Deciphering the Digital Tsunami: An In-depth Exploration of Big Data's Impact on Decision-Making, Innovation, and Business Transformation. *International Journal of Engineering and Advanced Technology Studies*, 10(1), 38–47.

Cruz T.M. 2020. Perils of data-driven equity: Safety-net care and big data's elusive grasp on health inequality. Big Data and Society, 7(1), 2053951720928097.

Davis O. and Carter E. 2021. Unveiling the Data Revolution: A Comprehensive Analysis of Big Data's Impact Across Industries. *Journal of Science and Technology*, 2(5), 40–47.

Din S.S.U., Ali M., Rashid U., Akbar, A.J. and Abid, M.K. 2023. Navigating an Optimization Path for Decision-Making in Management within The Big Data Environment of Chinese Public Hospitals. *International Journal of Information Systems and Computer Technologies*, 2(2), 61–77.

Dipietro L., Gonzalez-Mego P., Ramos-Estebanez C., Zukowski L.H., Mikkilineni R., Rushmore R.J. and Wagner T. 2023. The evolution of Big Data in neuroscience and neurology. *Journal of Big Data*, 10(1), 116.

Edison G. (2023). Transforming Medical Decision-Making: A Comprehensive Re view of AI's Impact on Diagnostics and Treatment. BULLET: J. Multidisiplin Ilmu, 2(4), 1121–33.

Furstenau L.B., Leivas P., Sott M.K., Dohan M.S., L´opez-Robles, J.R. Cobo, M.J. and Choo K.K.R. 2023. Big data in healthcare: Conceptual network structure, key challenges and opportunities. *Digital Communications and Networks*.

Ghaleb E.A., Dominic P.D., Muneer A. and Almohammedi A.A. 2022. Big Data in Healthcare Transformation: A short review. In 2022 International Conference on Decision Aid Sciences and Applications (DASA) (pp. 265–69). IEEE.

Hammami S., Durrah O., El-Maghraby L., Jaboob M., Kasim S. and Baalwi K. 2024. Understanding how big data awareness affects healthcare institution performance in Oman. In Artificial Intelligence, Big Data, Blockchain and 5G for the Digital Transformation of the Healthcare Industry (pp. 271–97). Academic Press.

Hassan S., Dhali M., Zaman F. and Tanveer M. 2021. Big data and predictive analytics in healthcare in Bangladesh: regulatory challenges. Heliyon, 7(6).

Johnson E. and Miller R. 2021. Harnessing the data revolution: big data's role in transforming industries. *Journal of Science and Technology*, 2(5), 32–39.

Korayim D., Chotia V., Jain G., Hassan S. and Paolone F. 2024. How can big data analytics create a competitive advantage in high-stake decision forecasting? The mediating role of organizational innovation. *Technological Forecasting and Social Change*, 199, 123040.

Liu C. and Li C. 2022. Mining the data goldmine: Big data's impact on AI algorithms and models. EPH-*International Journal of Business and Management Science*, 8(4), 1–4.

Omoyiola B.O. 2023. The social implications, risks, challenges and opportunities of big data. *Emerald Open Research*, 1(4).

Praveen S.P., Murali Krishna T.B., Anuradha C.H., Mandalapu S.R., Sarala P. and Sindhura S. 2022. A robust framework for handling health care information based on machine learning and big data engineering techniques. *International Journal of Healthcare Management*, 1–18.

Rao N.T., Bhattacharyya D. and Joshua E.S.N. 2022. An extensive discussion on utilization of data security and big data models for resolving healthcare problems. In Multi-chaos, fractal and multi-fractional artificial intelligence of different complex systems (pp. 311-24). Academic Press.

Secinaro S., Brescia V., Calandra D. and Biancone P. 2021. Data quality for health sector innovation and accounting management: A twenty-year bibliometric analysis. *Economia Aziendale Online*, 12(4), 407–31.

Shamshari A. and Najaf H. 2021. Mastering the data universe in AI : Big data's potential and challenges. *EPH-International Journal of Mathematics and Statistics*, 7(2), 1–4.

Thomson R. and Anderson J. 2021. Bridging the gap: Big data's influence on ai algorithms and models. *EPH-International Journal of Science and Engineering*, 7(4), 52–56.

Thomson R. and Anderson J. 2022. Big Data, Big Impact: How AI is Redefining Business Intelligence. *International Journal of Multidisciplinary Innovation and Research Methodology*, ISSN: 2960-2068, 1(1), 53–57.

Tunc-Abubakar T., Kalkan A. and Abubakar A.M. 2023. Impact of big data usage on product and process innovation: The role of data diagnosticity. Kybernetes, 52(9), 3178–96.

Wang W.Y.C. and Wang Y. 2020. Analytics in the era of big data: The digital transformations and value creation in industrial marketing. *Industrial Marketing Management*, 86, 12–15.

Weerasinghe K., Pauleen D., Taskin N. and Scahill S. 2023. Alignment of Big Data Perceptions Across Levels in Healthcare: The case of New Zealand. *Australasian Journal of Information Systems*, 27.

2

Artificial Intelligence and Machine Learning Approaches for Healthcare

Manjulata Badi[1*]

The COVID-19 pandemic has resulted in a significant change in the way that education is provided, moving away from traditional classroom instruction and toward extensive online training. The majority of modern technology apps contain machine learning algorithms. These algorithms are now indispensable to data science and our everyday lives, helping us in numerous ways. Artificial intelligence will become the most important disruptive technology-enabled civilization's facilitator as things improve. Without a doubt, machine learning methods and tools such as gradient-boosted-tree models (GBM), deep constitutional networks, generative adversarial networks (GAN), deep reinforcement learning (DRL), and others have propelled the revolution in the early detection of symptoms and the diagnosis and treatment of diseases in the pharmaceutical, healthcare, and related industries. Modern imaging methods such as MRI are crucial for the diagnosis of cancer and neurological disorders. This chapter will cover several medical datasets and resources that may be utilized to detect dementia using machine learning techniques. Recent advancements have increased the potential use of machine learning in cross-disciplinary study fields. The major goal of this chapter is to explain how machine learning may be used in the healthcare sector. There have already been significant advancements in machine learning, indicating its potential uses across several industries.

[1]   EEE Department, Alliance University, Bangalore, India
*   Corresponding author: mlbadi@gmail.com

Introduction

Artificial intelligence (AI) is a cutting-edge technology that has achieved success across various industries and has recently sparked academic interest. The COVID-19 pandemic poses an immediate threat to lives, disrupts social connections and hampers economic progress. Utilizing artificial intelligence, the latest scientific discipline, is essential in combating the epidemic. The two main contributions of this work are as follows. We enumerated the many uses of AI during the pandemic, including telemedicine services, material distribution, economic recovery, disinfection, vaccine development, patient diagnostics, elimination of potential viral carriers, and medical care We came to the conclusion that there were problems with multidimensional data, out-of-date algorithms, and a lack of systematicity in the technology during the pandemic in detail. It is vital to the progress of AI research and might establish a new standard for crises occurred (Ahmed et al., 2023).

Numerous instances of severe pneumonia were reported in Wuhan, in the province of Hubei, in December 2019. It was not determined what caused these occurrences. Samples from the lower respiratory tract were examined, and the novel severe acute respiratory syndrome coronavirus 2 (SARS-CoV-2) was shown to be the cause of this unique sickness. The coronavirus disease 2019 (COVID-19) pandemic has caused unanticipated financial losses as well as catastrophic global events that have escalated to the level of a global emergency (Acter et al., 2020). Globally, as of August 22, 2021, there were 4,432,648 fatalities and 211,993,378 confirmed cases. Moreover, insufficient evidence suggests that COVID-19 claims the lives of over 5,000 individuals worldwide every day.

The epidemic is still continuing strong almost a year and a half into its lifespan. These findings show that COVID-19 has grown out of control, and it is now important to consider how science could respond to such crises in the future. The study explores potential trajectories of SARS-CoV-2 infection and the impact of non-pharmaceutical interventions at the state level in the United States from 22 September 2020 through 28 February 2021 (Rajapaksha et al., 2021). It utilizes COVID-19 case and mortality data from 1 February 2020 to 21 September 2020, employing a deterministic SEIR (susceptible, exposed, infectious, and recovered) compartmental framework. According to the results of their experiment, widespread mask use (i.e., 95% of masks worn by people) would compare to two well-known broad-spectrum antiviral medications, Remdesivir (GS-5734) and Favipiravir (T-705). Among these medications were chloroquine, ribavirin, penciclovir, nitazoxanide, and nafamostat. Furthermore, their study demonstrates the effectiveness of remdesivir and chloroquine in preventing 2019-nCoV infection in vitro. Furthermore, Altan and Karasu (2020) created a hybrid model to recognize patients with coronavirus pneumonia from X-ray images by combining deep learning, the chaotic salp swarm approach (CSSA), and two-dimensional (2D) curvelet transformation.

The novel coronavirus disease, known as COVID-19, first appeared in Wuhan, China, in December 2019 and has since spread to almost every country in the world.

The severity of this epidemic reached an excessive level in no time (Patel and Kashyap, 2022). The outbreak forced several nations to impose lockdowns, close their borders, and practice social isolation in an effort to include supply chains, manufacturing, insurance, agriculture, transportation, and tourism (Wilder-Smith and Osman, 2020) and (Belhadi et al., 2021). The pandemic has had an unanticipated impact on global healthcare systems as well as the global economy.

Medical information has historically been mostly owned and accessed by healthcare professionals, such as doctors, radiologists, clinicians, and researchers, inside the closed ecosystem of isolated institutions that has historically constituted the healthcare system. There has only been one path for information to travel from healthcare provider to patient. But in the plurality of information-sharing connections including, many-to-many, one-to-many, and many-to-one, the one-to-one flow of information is being replaced (Euchi and Frifita, 2017). Under such circumstances, the bulk of coronavirus data obtained from clinical labs, hospitals, and the general public may not be reliable because the data is not monitored, is not kept on file, and is not collected in compliance with established guidelines (Wilder-Smith and Osman, 2020).

Reliable data is needed in order for the existing healthcare technology to deliver accurate and widely distributed services. Finally, tracking down or keeping an eye on infected people or their links raises a number of privacy problems. Healthcare organizations have been compelled to alter the present digital healthcare infrastructure in order to combat pandemic situations. Creating a more patient-centric and democratic digital healthcare environment is essential if we are to leverage digital platforms to combat COVID-19 and other pandemics. Recently, a lot of scholars have focused on using disruptive technologies—like blockchain and artificial intelligence transactions digitally (Pham et al., 2020). Blocks are connected chronologically by the miners, or nodes, that comprise the blockchain network.

As a result, blockchain facilitates the up to date maintenance of patient information, vaccination records, discharge summaries, and sample test results within a blockchain digital ledger. Through the use of self-executing contracts, or "smart contracts," these would enable the decentralized administration of healthcare information. Smart contracts are computer programs that carry out the specified terms of an agreement between parties when certain criteria are met inside the blockchain network (Djurovic and Janssen, 2018). Smart contracts built on blockchain technology may also automate processes related to audits, medical supply chain management, tracking epidemics, and remote patient monitoring. Furthermore, by training AI models collaboratively without sharing raw data, the federated learning paradigm has gained traction for healthcare applications to address data privacy and governance problems, security of health information (Mehta et al., 2020). Integrated blockchain and AI technologies have the potential to revolutionize the healthcare industry by extending the patient-centric approach (Khang et al., 2023). Spreading medicines and managing pandemic situations might be feasible ways to combat the coronavirus outbreak using a patient-centered approach. Then, we go over the products and useful uses of these cutting-edge technologies to support COVID-19 healthcare policies. The following are the article's contributions:

1. In theory, we reimagined the traditional healthcare paradigm with blockchain and AI for treating COVID-19 in a patient-centered manner.
2. In order to minimize the impact on healthcare, we used the existing public health efforts, such as the interchange of patient data, managing data for infection diagnosis, contact tracing, monitoring, and usage of the recommended decentralized, patient-centered frameworks.
3. We discussed the problems, solutions, and future research paths based on the study, all of which are anticipated to be highly beneficial to patients and the organizations that serve the healthcare sector.

This work is organized as follows: Section 2 covers relevant research and recent advancements in blockchain and AI-based healthcare solutions. In Section 3, the history of blockchain technology and AI are explained along with an overview of online medical services. Programs for Healthcare Management and Response Techniques during COVID-19 are used in Section 4. Section 5 concludes with future study topics and decentralized structure to assist pandemic healthcare measures.

Extra Effort

Blockchain and AI in Healthcare Systems

The most recent studies on blockchain technology and AI-based healthcare solutions are included in this area. A single point of failure, data manipulation, greater susceptibility to hostile cyberattacks, centralized authority, high maintenance costs, opaque databases, and costly data upkeep are the main dangers and problems associated with a traditional healthcare system. Researchers have created a plethora of blockchain-based solutions to address these issues. Using a blockchain-based server-client architecture network to store the hashed patient data allowed the developers (Jabarulla and Lee, 2021) to resolve security and privacy concerns. These server-client topologies, however, are vulnerable to a single point of failure. This offers a dispersed blockchain-based method for accessing patient and doctor data inside a healthcare institution. The removal of externalities is this system's main objective. In order to (Haleem et al., 2022) propose a framework AI-based healthcare systems need more data because of the ever-growing number of factors, complex structures, and quantity of information needed to provide accurate deep-learning solutions. Federated learning, which protects privacy while training locally stored data with local processing capacity, is one efficient distributed learning technique presented by Nguyen et al., 2021. By employing the federated learning technique, researchers may obtain a fair comprehension of patient data without disclosing any personal information about the patients (such as names, text messages, or prescription histories). Researchers can still obtain objective statistical insight even in cases where they do not have access to raw data, as they are frequently more interested in statistical outcomes than in data itself that provides a healthcare alliance.

Correlated Research Trends

The global COVID-19 pandemic outbreak in recent times has compelled a number of academics, professionals, and organizations to carry out comprehensive assessments with the aim of facilitating the creation of effective pandemic response and management. The clinical trials, facilitate medication treatment (Reddy and Badi, 2022). Disruptive technologies like blockchain and AI have made it possible to construct a number of healthcare applications that prioritize data protection, privacy, authenticity, and sharing at various levels, as well as COVID-19 data analysis investigated. The use of AI has been investigated for coronavirus medication development, forecasting, screening, and contact monitoring in this context.

The authors have reviewed the body of research on blockchain technology's potential to resolve complex issues brought on by the COVID-19 pandemic (Mbunge et al., 2021). The authors discussed significant blockchain applications on a platform built on blockchain technology to address problems brought up by the COVID-19 pandemic creating a cutting-edge conceptual architecture that combines blockchain technology and artificial intelligence to fight the COVID-19 epidemic. However, the only thing this article focuses on is a thorough assessment of current work on blockchain and artificial intelligence.

Based on the works listed above, we concluded that while many studies have focused on the current COVID-19 pandemic, they have only provided a rudimentary understanding of how to leverage blockchain and AI technology to combat COVID-19. As far as we are aware, no study has yet utilized blockchain and AI convergence to highlight the COVID-19 epidemic and its potential consequences in a decentralized, patient-centered framework. In order to achieve this goal, our new study has a higher potential to close research gaps and provide a detailed explanation of each layer and its roles within the conceptual framework.

Our research aims to give readers a basic, systematic framework for understanding the potential applications of blockchain technology with AI to support well-established public health strategies, using the envisioned patient-centric, decentralized approach.

General

The COVID-19 Pandemic and Digital Healthcare Services

Digital healthcare services facilitate more personalized pandemic preparedness and responses (Haleem et al., 2022). The phrase "digital health" is broad and encompasses mHealth, eHealth, blockchain, AI, big data, and the medical internet of things (MIoT). Despite the fact that telemedicine and telehealth have been available for a while, the healthcare sector has not adopted them as swiftly because of onerous regulations and inadequate funding models. Healthcare organizations were compelled to embrace the potential of digital technology to revolutionize healthcare delivery due to a spike of COVID-19 cases throughout the state (Gmunder et al., 2024).

Telemedicine can support diabetic patients in their battle against the COVID-19 pandemic, as has been shown in the past. To fight the coronavirus sickness, a variety of technologies like industry 4.0, multi-drone systems, and biosensors may be used (Kumar et al., 2021). The authors take the position that the cornerstone of pandemic management and response plans should be methodical. Their methodology demonstrates the efficient use of digital technology for pandemic preparedness, testing, monitoring, contact tracing, and quarantining in industrialized nations such as South Korea, Australia, Germany, Singapore, and Taiwan. Figure 2.1 highlights the responsibilities, difficulties, and the digital technologies used for the pandemic's management and response methods, as well as particular healthcare services and their challenges (Wang et al., 2021).

Patients: Anyone seeking medical assistance is considered a patient, and information about them is crucial for planning and responding to pandemics depicted in Figure 2.2.

Providers: These people or establishments include clinics, hospitals, physician offices, and laboratories that lead the battle against sickness by providing healthcare teams and researchers with access to health information.

Payers: A payer is a firm (like an insurance provider) that finances or reimburses the cost of prescription medications and medical services by paying people or organizations other than the patient. Payers also verify a patient's eligibility and handle payment transactions.

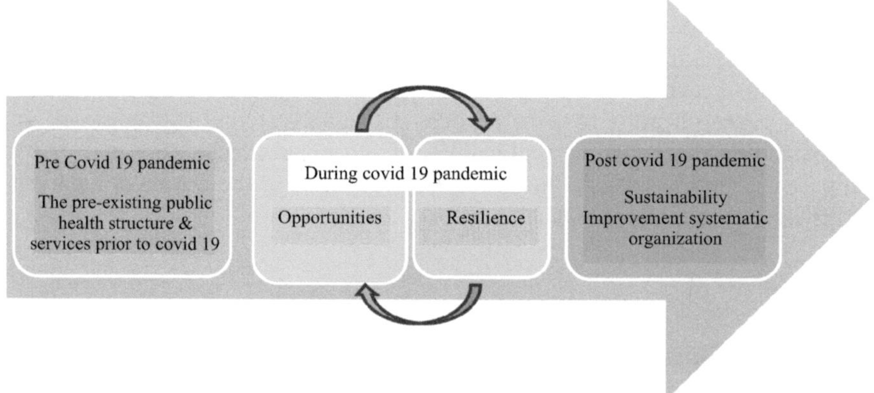

Fig. 2.1   Highlights the functions, difficulties, and digital technologies in pandemics

To give accurate information about the novel coronavirus spread or pandemic, health services need reliable data. Globally, a number of initiatives are being undertaken to promote a patient-centric culture by utilizing patient data, digital technology applications, and an increasing amount of research (Zou et al., 2022). The field of digital healthcare leveraging easier access to health data to track the

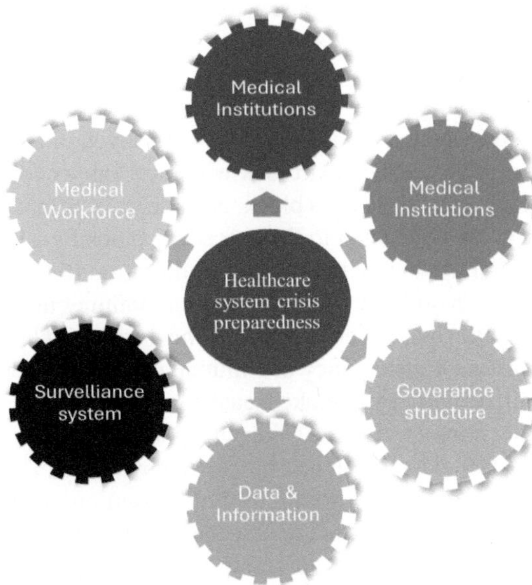

Fig. 2.2   COVID-19 health ecosystem

COVID-19 outbreak, identify high-risk patients, predict mortality, manage patient data, and combat pandemics and coronaviruses, is experiencing a significant rise in the adoption of disruptive technologies such as blockchain and AI. With AI, we can now filter through complicated factors and gain a thorough knowledge of cause and effect at the individual and population levels, something that was previously impossible. Companies are now able to comprehend the significance since blockchain makes it easier for the healthcare sector to move toward patient-driven and patient-mediated interoperability. This is crucial for the interchange of health information. In this study, we suggest a decentralized, patient-centered AI architecture for COVID-19 that is based on blockchain technology. We investigate the potential uses and applications of these interconnected technologies to enhance medical responses to the COVID-19 pandemic (Aman et al., 2021).

Artificial Intelligence and Blockchain Technologies

Blockchain is a cutting-edge and innovative technology that is mostly used in situations where centralization is an issue and anonymity is crucial. Blockchain is especially applicable to health data to emphasize sharing, dispersion, and encryption (Namasudra et al., 2021). The core ideas of a blockchain are decentralization and cryptographic hashing. Blockchain databases and data are accessible to all network users. Every member has access to the blockchain's contents since the network has produced a distributed, decentralized chain. The network's security is safeguarded by the consensus process. A consensus mechanism is a fault-tolerant method that helps all parties reach the required consensus on the state of the blockchain ledger at any given time by using a set of standards.

Nodes, blocks, and miners are the three main components of blockchain. In this context, a block is like a page in a record book since it has all or some portion of the most recent transaction data that hasn't been saved in any previous blocks. The blockchain advances to the next block whenever one is completed or mined. Every block, starting with the genesis block, is made up of data, a distinct none, and a hash value that, when connected to the preceding block by a hash label, forms a chain of blocks that inhibits any possibility of alteration in (Chi and Zhu, 2017). A blockchain network's nodes are in charge of maintaining network functionality and making sure that the data given is stored in the distributed ledger. Additionally, smart contracts increase transparency and mutual confidence between two parties by using blockchain technology to make it easier to create binding contracts that are enforceable. Transactions are tracked using an alphanumeric identification number that is exclusive to each participant in a blockchain network. This makes it simple for users of the distributed ledger to monitor and examine every transaction. The safe transactions of the smart contract reduce the likelihood of centralized authority involvement. Smart contracts that automate auditing procedures, provide time-limited access to distributed medical data, and enhance supply chain management development using the Ethereum Virtual Machine and Solidity platforms.

Blockchain technology has the potential to help stakeholders manage the massive amount of data that exists in the healthcare sector more effectively. Blockchain also creates private and safe protocols for the exchange of data in the healthcare sector. Healthcare applications include safe data management, transparent medical data storage and healthcare data privacy (Zaabar et al., 2021). These have shown the technology's tremendous potential because of blockchain's immutable and decentralized nature. AI technology is pervasive, however, it is essential for daily work. In addition, experts at Accenture forecast that between 2014 and 2021, the market for AI applications in healthcare will probably grow from $600 million to $6.6 billion. According to recent studies, AI-based ML and DL models are useful.

AI research benefits significantly from machine learning (ML), which offers great promise for identifying patterns and abnormalities in medical pictures' data. Then, by including this data into learning models, healthcare practitioners' decision-making is automated. Machine learning (ML) may be used, for instance, to create an automated facial recognition system that would identify body temperature and protect people against coronavirus infections. A deep learning architecture is made up of the several neural network layers that make up deep learning models (Singaravel et al., 2018). These layers are used to accept and train data samples, as well as to deliver training results. Here, the quantity of hidden layers regulates the DL architecture's depth.

Using labeled or unlabelled data samples that are linked to the hyper-parameter adjustments, supervised or unsupervised learning algorithms are employed to estimate the intended output. In order to recognize COVID-19 from chest radiography photos, AI built the COVID-Net framework utilizing visit duration, mortality, and risk of readmission. However, substantial, diverse, high-quality, private coronavirus datasets are needed for AI algorithms; these datasets might be shared by a number of healthcare facilities. Hence, to train datasets using a global AI model for identifying positive coronavirus infections, it is crucial to ensure acquisition of patient data related to COVID-19 cases. The researchers suggested federated learning frameworks as a solution to this data security issue, which would allow an AI model to be safely trained by examining a range of data stored at several places. Federated learning collects only the AI model parameters from several organizations while ensuring the security of the data. The fact that many federated learning algorithms rely on a single server raises security concerns about personal data. Researchers developed blockchain-based federated learning techniques to develop asynchronous collaborative AI models over a distributed network for a range of applications (Li et al., 2022). As a result, the federated learning, or DL, models based on blockchain technology operate without requiring a centralized server and refrain from directly transferring private patient information. To implement automated administration of "Cooperation" through the system is encouraged as blockchain allows the use of smart contracts to compensate users who provide data for the purpose of improving AI models. This decentralized approach to model training ensures the immutability of uploaded AI models and preserves privacy and security by calculating and recording the model quality on the blockchain. The patient-centric approach employs blockchain and artificial intelligence to solve COVID-19 issues while democratizing access to the ever-increasing volumes of patient data. The key components of AI and blockchain technology, which are vital in the fight against COVID-19, are depicted in Figure 2.3. Blockchain and artificial intelligence are driving innovation in digital healthcare, which has an immediate impact on providers and patients. Additionally, each of these technologies has a different level of technological complexity and ethical issues. Hence,combining them might help reduce COVID-19 by completely overhauling the current healthcare system to one that is patient-centered and decentralized. In summary, there are a number of benefits to addressing COVID-19 issues in healthcare through the application of blockchain and AI technologies.

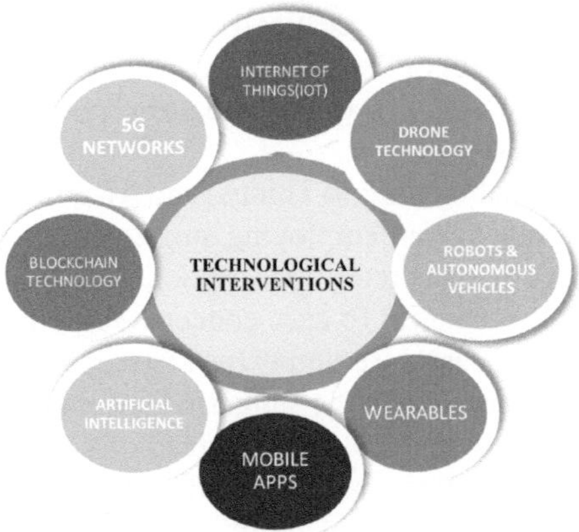

Fig. 2.3   Blockchain and AI technology in COVID-19

The patient-centric approach effectively integrates blockchain and AI to overcome COVID-19 challenges and democratizes the ever-increasing amounts of patient data. Figure 2.3 shows the salient features of blockchain and AI technologies that are essential in the fight against COVID-19. Digital healthcare is expanding faster because of blockchain and AI, which directly affects patients and providers. When these two technologies are combined, the present healthcare system may be fully transformed into a patient-centered, decentralized system, which may help minimize COVID-19. Additionally, the technological and ethical challenges raised by these two technologies range in degree. Blockchain and AI technologies should be used in healthcare to solve COVID-19 issues.

Programmes for Healthcare Management and Response Techniques During COVID-19

This section examines potential uses of the blockchain-based, AI-driven, patient-centric architecture as a result of the convergence of blockchain and AI technologies. Participants find it difficult to maintain their data, access to COVID-19 data is restricted, and standard healthcare is quite expensive. All of these are problems. Secure digital transaction monitoring, dispersed data access, and patient privacy are all guaranteed by the suggested patient-centric design.

Clinical Data Management and Information Sharing with a Patient-Centric Focus

Interoperability across healthcare participants is essential to the COVID-19 experiment. However, interoperability systems must adhere to national and international laws concerning data sharing, such as the Health Insurance Portability and Accountability Act (HIPAA) and the General Data Protection Regulation (GDPR). Patients need to be in control of their COVID-19 data in order to improve care standards and communication between caregivers and healthcare organizations. The patients must be the owners of their COVID personal health information (PHI), which may include blood oxygen levels, pulse rates, medication dosages, and scanned images of their bodies. Organizations like clinics, hospitals, or research centers that create or profit from data are not allowed to own personal health information (PHI).

Medical IoT (Medical Internet of Things) and AI-powered decentralized apps (dApps) built on the blockchain employing smart contracts allow medical data, like blood oxygen levels, heart rates, prescription dosages, and health history, to be collected in a private manner. To ease concerns regarding data tampering and forgeries, these gathered datasets are simply transferred to the suggested blockchain-based system. Furthermore, due to the suggested decentralized approach, doctors and patients may simply use telemedicine instead of visiting hospitals during the pandemic. The metadata is often not maintained in the blockchain. The precise data that is gathered from data sources is kept off-chain. Thus, using these techniques enables patients to provide their COVID-19 data while maintaining control over it and receiving token compensation. For instance, when patients handle health data using blockchain technology, they may safely gather, share, give, sell, and manage their PHRs. Patients may benefit from using their COVID data to train an AI model that will use their X-ray or CT scan data to provide a quicker and more accurate diagnosis, or to forecast an epidemic. The patient-centric approach maintains participant confidence and helps to preserve patient privacy by promoting transparency in data storage and exchange. Smart contracts can help the blockchain promote security for clinical trial data.

Decentralized Contact Tracing

Contact-tracing software is an essential digital health technology supporting the efforts to combat the COVID-19 epidemic. Numerous technologies, including GPS, Wi-Fi, Bluetooth, mobile apps, social networks, contact data, network-based APIs, and quick response (QR) codes for smartphones, can be used to offer contact tracings. Due to security and privacy issues, it is still difficult to identify those who have been infected with viruses. By weighing the needs of public health and privacy and data analysis, the decentralized, patient-centric solution built on blockchain and AI can allay these worries. Using blockchain technology, individuals may securely exchange their personal information with public health organizations, such as government health authorities or commercial databases endorsed by the government, without disclosing their identities. This might be useful in warning anyone who comes into contact with coronavirus-positive patients without disclosing any further personal information or medical records. Additionally, by running the collected data through an AI model, clusters and hotspots may be located. The results of the AI model may be a crucial instrument for encouraging a more responsible economic recovery without increasing the number of cases. Researchers are using blockchain technology to provide COVID-19 vaccination recipients digital passports that are safeguarded. Public health professionals just need to certify these health certificates in order to validate an individual's condition.

Outbreak Prognosis

This data is used by AI models to evaluate the risks associated with the sickness and its ability to spread. AI may be used to determine which nations and individuals are most at risk. Additionally, it has the ability to forecast the quantity of positive situations, which enables the proactive adoption of pertinent policies. By analyzing how people use their phones and determining the magnitude of the epidemic, AI can also stop the spread of COVID-19. This assessment takes into account the possibility that a COVID patient's or deceased person's phone use pattern may change since the phone may be unused or utilized by a family member. By examining the wireless data, these modifications in patterns enabled people to model and anticipate their phone usage histories by using machine learning to identify their distinct, erratic mobile behaviors. With the use of DL, they were also able to precisely assess how mobile phone apps were being used, including strange calling patterns and inactive phone service. Deploying blockchain-enabled dApps on patients' mobile devices specifically aids in tracking and predicting the global spread of the viral infection by anonymously preserving patient data.

Coronavirus Analysis and Detection

By using ML and DL algorithms, AI enables an automated decision-making system that facilitates the development of a unique, affordable diagnosis solution for COVID-19 cases. Medical professionals may be able to recognize COVID-19 infractions and symptoms, for instance, by utilizing AI-powered facial recognition to detect a person's mask-wearing status and facial temperature. AI analyzes images from CT, MRI, and chest X-ray scans to enable automated diagnosis of the infected cases. To effectively discover COVID-19 thoracic CT characteristics, the scientists developed a detection strategy that merged two- and three-dimensional DL approaches with pre-existing AI models. This was done by distinguishing between the traits associated with COVID-19 and influenza pneumonia. The study indicates that viral pneumonia may also occur. To identify features and distinguish between influenza A viral pneumonia, COVID-19 viral pneumonia, and healthy persons, the researchers looked at a series of lung CT images. In another study, chest X-ray radiographs were evaluated using models based on convolutional neural networks to determine whether individuals had viral pneumonia brought on by the COVID-19 virus. The cases listed above indicate the importance of coronavirus data. To maintain privacy, the medical data that is used to train the AI models is split and kept on many servers. Consequently, it is challenging to get a good result across populations. Federated learning's decentralized, patient-centered design may make it possible.

Emergency Assistance and Insurance

Widespread lockdowns and social segregation laws sometimes result in COVID pandemic conditions with significant hazards, including the potential for disruption of the healthcare delivery system and long-term effects on people' physical health like supply chain management, pharmaceutical supplies, information sharing and data management technology, and medically mandated social services. The present healthcare system's centralization, opacity, and reliance on labor-intensive paper-based procedures are its primary culprits.

By replacing conventional paper-based rules with a method does away with the need for intermediaries and processing delays. In addition to lowering operational risk, the smart contract streamlines complex applications to speed up the loan and insurance approval process. Many parties, including governments, pharmaceutical corporations, and regulatory organizations, create and implement policy agreements on blockchain networks in order to deliver timely, dependable, and scalable solutions within patient-centric healthcare consortia. In addition, the patient is increasingly the center of attention for the revenue cycle and other operational aspects of healthcare. As a result, patients now have a choice in hospitals, payers, and pharmaceutical firms they engage with. Additionally, these providers must offer service standards that are comparable to those seen in retailing.

Supply Chain Management

The healthcare provider and the supply chain play a crucial role in ensuring patient care and safety. Due to rapid changes in consumer purchase habits, transportation routes, and supply shortages, the COVID-19 pandemic's shockwave caused disturbances in the worldwide supply system. Panic purchasing, for instance, increased demand for household necessities. Because there is a lack of integration and interest alignments in the healthcare supply chain, COVID-19 has brought particular attention to the problems associated with managing the supply chains for medications and medical equipment. Therefore, in order to address new issues brought on by the ongoing worldwide pandemic and control the flow of medical supplies, it is vital that the current supply chain system be completely reconstructed.

Using blockchain technology, this decentralized, patient-centric approach makes it possible to create a supply chain ecosystem that is more reliable, robust, and completely integrated. Here, the blockchain takes into account a variety of stakeholders in an anonymous manner, with aspects such as better customer service and care being offered that serve as unifying factors. Through the deployment of blockchain-enabled dApps, patients will be connected to the system data. Thus, provenance, auditability, and transparency are supported by keeping unchangeable records of data logs. Supply chain organizations may move items quickly, reliably, and securely from the source to the destination by utilizing a blockchain.

Conclusion

The pandemic management services released a theoretical framework for a patient-centered, decentralized healthcare system that integrates blockchain technology and artificial intelligence (AI) to combat the coronavirus outbreak. There are four potential uses for the decentralized, patient-centered design that has been suggested. It first enhances communication between payers, providers, governments, pharmaceutical companies, and researchers—all parties involved on the healthcare platform. Second, patients securely keep their COVID-19 medical data and control their personal information on patient-centric blockchain systems.

References

Acter T., Uddin N., Das J., Akhter A., Choudhury T.R. et al., 2020. Evolution of severe acute respiratory syndrome coronavirus 2 (SARS-CoV-2) as coronavirus disease 2019 (COVID-19) pandemic: A global health emergency. *Science of the Total Environment*, 730, 138996.

Ahmed S., Yong J. and Shrestha A. 2023. The Integral Role of Intelligent IoT System, Cloud Computing, Artificial Intelligence, and 5G in the User-Level Self-Monitoring of COVID-19. Electronics, 12(8), 1912.

Aman A.H.M., Hassan W.H., Sameen S., Attarbashi Z.S., Alizadeh M. et al., 2021. IoMT amid COVID-19 pandemic: Application, architecture, technology, and security. *Journal of Network and Computer Applications*, 174, 102886.

Belhadi A., Kamble S., Jabbour C.J.C., Gunasekaran A., Ndubisi N.O. et al., 2021. Manufacturing and service supply chain resilience to the COVID-19 outbreak: Lessons learned from the automobile and airline industries. *Technological forecasting and social change*, 163, 120447.

Chi L. and Zhu X. 2017. Hashing techniques: A survey and taxonomy. *ACM Computing Surveys (Csur)*, 50(1), 1–36.

Djurovic M. and Janssen A. 2018. The formation of blockchain-based smart contracts in the light of contract law. *European Review of Private Law*, 26(6).

Euchi J. and Frifita S. 2017. Hybrid metaheuristic to solve the "one-to-many-to-one" problem: Case of distribution of soft drink in Tunisia. *Management Decision*, 55(1), 136–55.

Gmunder K.N., Ruiz J.W., Franceschi D. and Suarez M.M. 2024. Demographics associated with US healthcare disparities are exacerbated by the telemedicine surge during the COVID-19 pandemic. *Journal of Telemedicine and Telecare*, 30(1), 64–71.

Haleem A., Javaid M., Singh R.P. and Suman R. 2022. Medical 4.0 technologies for healthcare: Features, capabilities, and applications. *Internet of Things and Cyber-Physical Systems*, 2, 12–30.

Jabarulla M.Y. and Lee H.N. 2021. A blockchain and artificial intelligence-based, patient-centric healthcare system for combating the COVID-19 pandemic: *Opportunities and applications in Healthcare* (Vol. 9, No. 8, p. 1019). MDPI.

Khang A., Rana G., Tailor R.K. and Abdullayev V. (Eds.). 2023. Data-Centric AI Solutions and Emerging Technologies in the Healthcare Ecosystem.

Kumar A., Sharma K., Singh H., Naugriya S.G., Gill S.S. et al., 2021. A drone-based networked system and methods for combating coronavirus disease (COVID-19) pandemic. *Future Generation Computer Systems*, 115, 1–19.

Li D., Luo Z. and Cao B. 2022. Blockchain-based federated learning methodologies in smart environments. *Cluster Computing*, 25(4), 2585–99.

Mbunge E., Akinnuwesi B., Fashoto S.G., Metfula A.S., Mashwama P. et al., 2021. A critical review of emerging technologies for tackling COVID-19 pandemic. *Human Behavior and Emerging Technologies*, 3(1), 25–39.

Mehta S., Grant K. and Ackery A. 2020. Future of blockchain in healthcare: Potential to improve the accessibility, security and interoperability of electronic health records. *BMJ Health & Care Informatics*, 27(3).

Namasudra S., Deka G.C., Johri P., Hosseinpour M. and Gandomi A.H. et al., 2021. The revolution of blockchain: State-of-the-art and research challenges. *Archives of Computational Methods in Engineering*, 28, 1497–1515.

Nguyen D.C., Ding M., Pham Q.V., Pathirana P.N., Le L.B., Seneviratne, A. et al., 2021. Federated learning meets blockchain in edge computing: Opportunities and challenges. *IEEE Internet of Things Journal*, 8(16), 12806–12825.

Patel R.K. and Kashyap M. 2022. Automated diagnosis of COVID stages from lung CT images using statistical features in 2-dimensional flexible analytic wavelet transform. *Biocybernetics and Biomedical Engineering*, 42(3), 829–41.

Pham Q.V., Nguyen D.C., Huynh-The T., Hwang W.J., Pathirana P.N. et al., 2020. Artificial intelligence (AI) and big data for coronavirus (COVID-19) pandemic: A survey on the state-of-the-arts. *IEEE access*, 8, 130820–130839.

Rajapaksha R.N.U., Wijesinghe M.S.D., Thomas T.K., Jayasooriya S.P., Gunawardana B.I. et al., 2021. An Extended Susceptible-Exposed-Infected-Recovered (SEIR) Model with Vaccination for Predicting the COVID-19 Pandemic in Sri Lanka. medRxiv, 1–33.

Reddy D. and Badi M. (2022). Non-Contact Temperature Measurement Applicable for Covid-19. *Journal of Advancement in Electronics Design*, 5(2), 33–46.

Singaravel S., Suykens J. and Geyer P. 2018. Deep-learning neural-network architectures and methods: Using component-based models in building-design energy prediction. *Advanced Engineering Informatics*, 38, 81–90.

Wang Q., Su M., Zhang M. and Li R. 2021. Integrating digital technologies and public health to fight Covid-19 pandemic: Key technologies, applications, challenges and outlook of digital healthcare. *International Journal of Environmental Research and Public Health*, 18(11), 6053.

Wilder-Smith A. and Osman S. 2020. Public health emergencies of international concern: a historic overview. Journal of travel medicine, 27(8), taaa227.

Zaabar B., Cheikhrouhou O., Jamil F., Ammi M., Abid M. et al., 2021. HealthBlock: A secure blockchain-based healthcare data management system. *Computer Networks*, 200, 108500.

Zou K.H., Salem L.A. and Ray A. (Eds.). 2022. Real-World Evidence in a Patient-Centric Digital Era. CRC Press.

3

Predictive Analytics Tools and Techniques for Disease Prevention and Early Detection in Healthcare Sector

Prakash Kuppuswamy,[1*] *M. Mohan,*[1] *Sayed QY Al Khalidi*[2] and *Vijaya Varshini Prakash*[3]

Predictive analytics has emerged as a powerful tool in healthcare, revolutionizing the way we approach patient care. The use of advanced data analysis techniques to forecast future outcomes and trends based on historical data enables healthcare providers to make better decisions and take proactive measures. Predictive analytics methods perform a key role in extracting respected insights from data sets and then making predictions about future events. In particular, prediction algorithms have immense potential for the prevention and early detection of diseases. By leveraging healthcare data and advanced analytics techniques, these algorithms enable timely interventions, personalized medicine, resource optimization, and cost savings. Prevention and early detection of diseases are critical aspects of healthcare that can significantly improve patient outcomes and costs. With advancements in technology and the availability of healthcare data, prediction algorithms have emerged as powerful tools for identifying individuals at risk of developing various diseases. In this article, we will explore the use of prediction algorithms in prevention and

[1] Computer Science Engineering, SRM University, Delhi NCR, India
[2] Department of Information Technology, King Khalid University, Abha, KSA
[3] Palaniappa College of Arts & Science, Bharathiyar University, T.N., India
* Corresponding author: prakashcnet@gmail.com

early detection, their benefits, challenges, and best practices, and also delve into the world of predictive analytics tools and methods, exploring their capabilities, benefits, and best practices in the healthcare industry.

Introduction

Prediction algorithms leverage techniques from machine learning, statistical modeling, and data mining to analyze healthcare information and categorize patterns that can be used to predict the risk of developing diseases (Hossain M.E. et al., 2019; Ishaq A. et al., 2021; Rajula H.S. et al., 2020). Prediction methods can integrate various data types, containing demographic statistics, medical information, genetic data, and lifestyle factors, to develop accurate threat models (Chatterjee A. et al., 2020; Lee A. et al., 2019; Kyrou I. et al., 2020). The method of predictive analytics refers to the use of data, machine learning prototypes, and statistical methods to forecast imminent results and trends (Seyedan M. and Mafakheri F., 2020; Bharadiya J.P., 2023). By analyzing historical data patterns, predictive analytics seeks to recognize relationships and patterns that can be used to identify future predictions (Sheng J. et al., 2021; Alam A. and Mohanty A., 2022; Zhao L., 2021). Analytics models, as mentioned in Figure 3.1 are an essential tool for extracting insight and value from data. They help businesses make informed decisions, predict future outcomes, optimize operations, and gain a competitive edge (Khang A. et al., 2023). There are various types of analytics models, each serving a specific purpose. In this article, we will explore some of the most common types of analytics models and their applications (Khang A. et al., 2023; Souza P.C. et al., 2021).

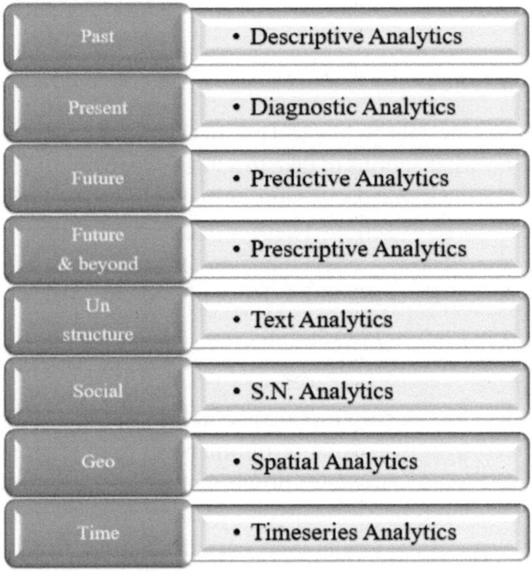

Fig. 3.1   Analytics types

Descriptive Analytics

The descriptive models focus on past events' data to access insights into earlier trials and tendencies. They provide a comprehensive understanding of what has happened and why. Descriptive models include techniques such as data visualization, reporting, and basic statistical analysis. These models are useful for tracking key performance indicators (KPIs) and understanding the overall state of a business (Ravanelli M. et al., 2021).

Diagnostic Analytics

Diagnostic analytics models aim to identify the causes of past events or trends. They dig deeper into the data to uncover why certain outcomes occurred. Diagnostic models use techniques such as root cause analysis, correlation analysis, and hypothesis testing. By understanding the underlying factors that drive specific results, businesses can make adjustments to improve performance (Burger J. et al., 2022).

Predictive Analytics

Predictive analytics models focus on forecasting future outcomes based on historical patterns and trends. These models use statistical algorithms, machine learning techniques, and data mining to make predictions. Predictive models can help businesses anticipate customer behavior, identify trends, and optimize processes. They are widely used in customer churn prediction, demand forecasting, and fraud detection, among other applications (Low D.M. et al., 2020; Seyedan M. and Mafakheri F. 2020).

Prescriptive Analytics

Prescriptive analytics models go beyond predicting future outcomes. They provide recommendations on what actions to take to achieve specific objectives. Prescriptive models use optimization algorithms, simulation techniques, and decision analysis to suggest the best course of action. These models help businesses make informed decisions in areas such as supply chain management, resource allocation, and pricing optimization (Lepenioti K. et al., 2020; Hoyos W. et al., 2023).

Text Analytics

Text analytics models focus on extracting useful information from unorganized text information, such as buyer assessments, public blogs, or documents. These models use techniques like natural language processing (NLP), sentiment analysis, and topic modeling. Text analytics models can help businesses understand customer feedback, identify emerging trends, and extract insights from large volumes of textual data (Kang Y. et al., 2020).

Social Network Analytics

Social network analytics models analyze social connections and interactions to gain insights into social structures, influences, and dynamics. These models are used to understand how individuals or groups influence each other's behaviors, spread information, and form communities. Social network analytics is crucial in marketing, brand management, and social media campaigns, where understanding the network effects is paramount (Ahmed W. et al., 2022).

Spatial Analytics

Spatial analytics models analyze data with geographic or spatial components. They help businesses uncover patterns, relationships, and trends in data related to a specific location. These models are used in urban planning, logistics optimization, site selection, and environmental analysis. Spatial analytics combines traditional statistical techniques with geographic information systems (GIS) to provide valuable insights (Park S. et al., 2020).

Time Series Analytics

Time series analytics models analyze data that is poised over time to identify patterns, trends, and seasonality. These models are used for forecasting future values and understanding long-term trends. Time series models are widely used in finance, stock market analysis, sales forecasting, and resource planning (Feng M. et al., 2019; Ray S. et al., 2021).

These are just a few examples of the different types of analytical models. Each type serves a specific purpose and has its own unique techniques and methodologies. Depending on the business needs and available data, organizations can employ one or more models to make data-driven decisions to optimize processes (Nath P. et al., 2021; Athiyarath S. et al., 2020). With advanced analytics techniques, healthcare organizations can make more accurate predictions and data-driven decisions. This can lead to improved patient outcomes, better resource management, and cost savings. However, it is crucial to address the challenges, such as data privacy and ethical considerations, when implementing predictive analytics systems. With ongoing advancements in technology and increasing adoption, predictive analytics is set to play an even more crucial role in healthcare in the coming years (Ogbuke N.J. et al., 2022; Tursunbayeva A. et al., 2022). The prevention and early detection of diseases using prediction algorithms offer several benefits, as shown in Figure 3.2.

- *Timely intervention:* By identifying individuals at high risk of developing a disease, prediction algorithms enable healthcare professionals to intervene proactively. Early detection allows for prompt treatment, lifestyle modifications, and preventive measures that can potentially delay or even prevent the onset of the disease (Ngiam K.Y. and Khor W. 2019; Porsteinsson A.P. et al., 2021).

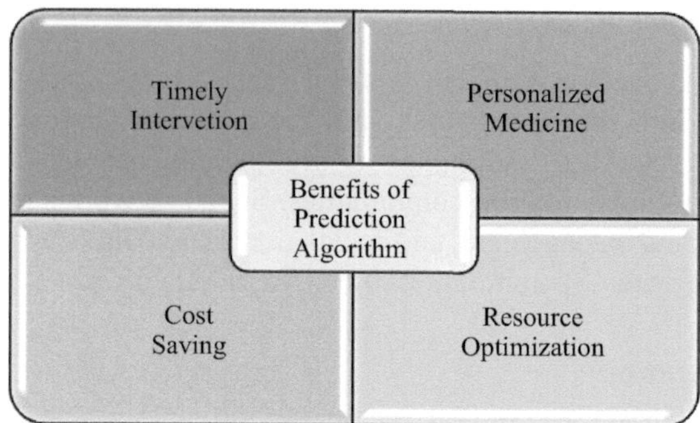

Fig. 3.2   Benefits of prediction algorithm

- *Personalized medicine:* Prediction algorithms take individual characteristics and risk factors into account, enabling the delivery of personalized healthcare interventions. Tailoring prevention strategies to an individual's specific risk profile enhances the effectiveness and efficiency of healthcare treatments (Paulus J.K. and Kent D.M., 2020).
- *Resource optimization:* By targeting interventions and screenings to individuals at high risk, prediction algorithms optimize the allocation of healthcare resources. This improves resource management, reduces unnecessary screenings, and ensures that preventive measures are directed to those who would benefit the most (Fitzgerald R.C. et al., 2022).
- *Cost savings:* Prevention and early detection lead to cost savings in healthcare. By identifying diseases at an early stage, treatment can be less invasive and less expensive. Additionally, preventing the onset or progression of chronic diseases reduces the long-term healthcare costs associated with managing these conditions (Park Y.J. et al., 2020).

Related Studies

Several key challenges face the healthcare industry, including electronic record management, data integration, and computer-assisted diagnosis and prediction. Healthcare costs must be reduced, and personalized healthcare must be implemented. Predictive analytics in healthcare is emerging as a transformative tool that can be used to provide proactive and preventative treatments. An overview of deep learning techniques and tools in practice as well as deep learning applications in healthcare is provided, and it describes the framework for deep learning data analysis in clinical decision making. (Muniasamy A. et al., 2020). It is essential to take proper care of health data since it contains complex data and information, such as the patient's past information and caregiver, as well as the patient's medical condition. A leak of this private information can result in bullying, higher insurance premiums, and job loss due to medical history. It is therefore extremely important to protect, maintain, and trust the information. In addition, government regulations and ethics committees demand that healthcare data be secure and privacy-protected. Also, it identifies challenges, and examines requirements. Regulations, ethical guidelines, and domain-specific needs are explored in this research work. Additionally, it examines machine learning algorithms that can be used to calculate precision health data in a secure and privacy-preserving manner, as well as their applications to relevant health applications (Thapa and Camtepe, 2021).

The incorporation of Artificial intelligence (AI) and machine learning in occupational intelligence has resulted in a variety of tendencies and possibilities. These state-of-the-art technologies have transformed the way traders analyze data, obtain insights, and mark conversant choices. A notable development is the emergence of predictive analytics, which enables companies to discover concealed patterns, spot growth opportunities, enhance business processes, and ultimately drive their achievements through well-informed decisions. AI-powered chatbots and virtual assistants are another trend. Machine learning and AI offer a wide range of business intelligence opportunities. Business can enhance developments, minimize costs, and identify potential new revenue schemes through independent variable studies, inconsistency identification, customer demand, and flexible pricing, among other strategies (Maheshwari and Gautam, 2021). In exploring contemporary management topics and the global challenges brought about by the COVID-19 pandemic, a range of analytics techniques can offer valuable guidance to scholars. In this Methodology Corner, we offer an overview of innovative approaches to studying big data analytics and their potential for examining present-day organizational concerns more effectively. This article offers insights into descriptive/diagnostic, predictive and prescriptive analytics and their application to COVID-19-related global crises (Sheng J. et al., 2021).

Predictive analytics based on machine learning have proven to be effective in the healthcare sector. Medical data can be analyzed using these techniques to extract meaningful insights. It is possible to reduce the mortality rate and eliminate expensive healthcare costs by predicting diseases at the preliminary stage. A summary has been provided to give information on chronic diseases, their biological correlates, as well as how ML algorithm-based predictive analytics can be used to predict chronic diseases early in the healthcare sector (Hegde, S.K. and Mundada M.R. 2022). An investigation of how predictive analytics and machine learning can be used in healthcare to prevent disease is explored in this research study. These technologies are transforming disease identification, diagnosis, and treatment by analyzing vast amounts of patient data, leading to more effective preventive measures. Machine learning and predictive analytics are making a significant impact in several key areas, according to the findings of this study. By identifying subtle patterns in medical records, lab results, genetic information, and imaging data, machine learning algorithms can facilitate early detection and diagnosis (Ibrahim M.S. and Saber S. 2023).

The majority of research studies focus on describing specific disease findings without discussing methodology or evaluating the findings. This study provides a comprehensive guide to predicting various diseases, identifying them in the past, present, and future.

Significance of Research

In the healthcare sector, the use of predictive analytics has the potential to revolutionize patient care, improve operational efficiency, and enhance decision-making processes. The need for predictive analytics in healthcare arises from the increasing complexity and vastness of healthcare data. With the significant usage and benefits of electronic health records (EHRs) and other digital health technologies, healthcare organizations have access to an ever-growing wealth of patient information. However, harnessing this information and turning it into actionable insights can be a daunting task without the help of analytics.

In the field of healthcare, predictive analytics plays a crucial role in anticipating and averting negative outcomes. By analyzing historical data, healthcare providers can identify patterns and risk factors associated with medical errors, hospital-acquired infections, medication errors, and other adverse events. This allows them to proactively implement targeted interventions and protocols to mitigate these risks, resulting in improved patient safety and outcomes. Another important application of predictive analytics is in disease diagnosis and prognosis. By assessing patient data such as previous diagnostics, symptoms, medical image reports, and genomics, predictive models can be developed to identify and predict diseases at an early stage. For example, predictive analytics can help detect signs of certain types of cancer or chronic diseases before they manifest clinically. This enables healthcare providers to initiate early interventions and personalized treatment plans, potentially saving lives and reducing healthcare costs.

In addition to predictive models for individual patients, healthcare organizations can also utilize predictive analytics for population health management. By analyzing data on a large scale, such as demographic information, socio-economic factors, environmental data, and healthcare utilization patterns, public health agencies and medical professionals can categorize potential-risk populations and design battered interferences to progress to complete health results. For example, predictive analytics can help predict the spread of infectious diseases, identify areas with high prevalence rates of chronic illnesses, and allocate resources accordingly. Operational efficiency is another area where predictive analytics can bring significant improvements to healthcare organizations. By analyzing historical data on patient flow, resource utilization, appointment scheduling, and staffing levels, hospitals and clinics can optimize their processes and resources to reduce wait times, improve patient access, and improve complete functioning productivity. This can lead to patient appraisal levels and also budget reserves for healthcare organizations.

- Improved patient care
- Health management
- Personalized Treatment
- Identify risk level of patient
- Chronic Disease Management
- Healthcare track

Prediction algorithms heavily rely on the availability of high-quality and comprehensive healthcare data. Challenges related to data collection, data privacy, data interoperability, and data biases can impact the accuracy and reliability of predictive models. Many prediction models, such as deep learning algorithms, are well-thought-out "black-box" models, making it challenging to realize the intellectual behind their prophecies. It raises ethical considerations such as informed consent, data privacy, fairness, and transparency. It is crucial to address these ethical challenges to ensure that predictive models are used responsibly and ethically.

Data Analytics vs. Predictive Analytics

Data analytics and predictive analytics are two valuable tools in the field of data science that empower establishments to expand perceptions and mark cognizant verdicts based on their data. While they both share the common goal of extracting insights from data, there are distinct differences between data analytics tools and predictive analytics tools. Here, we will explore these differences in detail.

Data analytics tools are designed to analyze historical data and discover patterns, trends, and correlations within the dataset. These tools are primarily focused on describing and summarizing the data to extract useful insights. The main goal of data analytics is to answer questions such as "What happened?" or "Why did it happen?"

One of the primary features of data analytics tools is the ability to perform descriptive statistics. Descriptive statistics provide summary information about the data, such as the mean, median, mode, standard deviation, and other statistical measures. These statistics give organizations a better understanding of their data distribution and help identify outliers or anomalies. Data analytics tools also provide various visualization capabilities to present insights in a data visualization facility that can be easy to understand. Data appearances such as graphic representations, Gantt charts, and heat maps are frequently used to characterize patterns and trends found in the data set. These visualizations help stakeholders to interpret the results easily and identify actionable insights.

On the other hand, predictive analytics tools go beyond historical analysis and aim to forecast future outcomes based on patterns and trends in the data. Predictive models consist of using previous and past data, as well as, statistical methods to create predictions and assess the likelihood of certain events or outcomes. The primary question that predictive analytics seeks to answer is "What is likely to happen?"

Predictive analytics utilizes advanced algorithms and machine learning techniques to train models on past data and create predictions on new, unseen data. These models are developed to identify relationships and patterns in the data and use them to make future predictions. Applying relevant training data set modules to predictive analytics tools leads to producing effectiveness and accuracy of prediction results. In addition to identifying patterns, predictive analytics also considers various factors and variables that can impact the outcome. These factors can include external variables, seasonality, market trends, and other relevant data sources. By considering multiple variables, predictive analytics can provide more accurate forecasts and assist organizations in making better-informed decisions.

Another key aspect of predictive analytics is the ability to determine the strength and significance of relationships between variables. Through techniques like regression analysis, predictive analytics tools can quantify the impact of different factors on the predicted outcome. This helps organizations understand which variables have the most significant influence and plan their strategies accordingly. While both data analytics and predictive analytics tools are vital for data-driven decision-making, they differ in their objectives and focus. Data analytics tools primarily aim to gain insights from historical data by describing and summarizing the data, while predictive analytics tools focus on understanding patterns and making predictions about future outcomes.

Data analytics helps organizations understand what happened in the past, while predictive analytics empowers organizations to anticipate what may happen in the future. By leveraging both of these tools, organizations can harness the power of data to gain a holistic view of their procedures and achieve data-driven choices that lead to success. In Table 3.1. we summarize the differences between data analytics and predictive analytics for a better understanding.

Table 3.1   Comparison of data and predictive analytics

Basic comparison of Data analytics and Predictive analytics	
FORM	
An analysis of data used in business is considered a form of 'general' analytics.	Using predictive analytics, businesses can predict the outcome of future events.
STRUCTURE	
The purpose of data analytics is to collect and analyze data in general.	Statistical modeling, analysis, and monitoring are the steps involved in predictive analytics, along with defining a project and collecting data.
DATA	
Data Analytics is performed using clean data obtained from churned raw data.	Predictive Analytics can be done with clean data.
SEQUENCE	
Analyzing data consists of several steps: collecting the data, inspecting it, cleaning and transforming it, and analyzing the results.	In predictive analytics, data is modeled, the model is trained, and the outcome is predicted and forecasted.
OUTCOME	
Data Analytics may or may not lead to predictive results ; it depends on the business case.	Statistical models allow us to test assumptions and hypotheses before creating an exact future model based on predictive analysis.
USAGE	
In addition to uncovering hidden patterns and finding correlations, data analytics can be used by businesses to learn more about customer preferences and market trends.	Predictive analytics helps answer questions such as "What will happen if demand goes down? What will be the risk of losing money in a new business enterprise?"

The Role of Predictive Analytics in Healthcare

Now let's explore some of the key applications of prediction algorithms in preventing and detecting diseases.

Cancer prediction

Prediction algorithms can analyze various factors, such as family history, genetic markers, lifestyle choices, and environmental exposures, to assess an individual's risk of developing different types of cancer. These algorithms enable targeted screening programs, genetic counseling, and early interventions.

Cardiovascular disease prediction

Prediction algorithms can analyze features such as patient age, cholesterol, blood pressure, consumption of alcohol, smoking, and family heritage data to estimate an individual's risk of increasing cardiovascular diseases, such as heart disease and stroke. This information enables the implementation of preventive strategies, including lifestyle modifications and medication management.

Diabetes prediction

Prediction algorithms can analyze risk factors such as body mass index (BMI), glucose levels, insulin resistance, and genetic markers to calculate the risk of diabetes. Early identification of individuals at risk allows for lifestyle interventions and closer monitoring to prevent or delay the onset of the disease.

Infectious disease prediction

Prediction algorithms can analyze various data sources, including social media, climate data, and demographic information, to predict the risk of infectious disease outbreaks. These algorithms can aid in early detection, response planning, resource allocation, and public health interventions.

Drug Discovery and Development

Another significant benefit of the prediction analytics module is to identify and involve drug discovery and development. By analyzing vast amounts of biological and chemical data, algorithms can identify potential drug candidates with higher success rates, reducing the time and cost involved in the development of new medications.

Predictive Analytics Tools

Predictive analytics tools are essential in today's data-driven world. They empower businesses to make informed decisions, anticipate trends, and gain a competitive edge. Here, we will compare several popular predictive analytics tools, examining their features, functionalities, and strengths.

IBM Watson Studio

- Watson Studio offers a wide-ranging set of tools for data science and machine learning.
- It offers a user-friendly interface, allowing both technical and non-technical users to work with data effectively.
- Key features include AI model building, automated ML, data preparation, and deployment capabilities.
- It integrates with various data sources and provides advanced visualization options.
- However, the complexity and learning curve may be challenging for novice users.

Microsoft Azure Machine Learning

- Azure ML is a cloud-based system that allows users to build, deploy, and manage machine learning models at scale.
- It provides a drag-and-drop interface, simplifying the data science process.
- The tool provides a wide range of pre-built algorithms and supports custom model creation.
- Azure ML integrates seamlessly with other Microsoft products and services.
- However, the pricing structure may be a deterrent for small businesses.

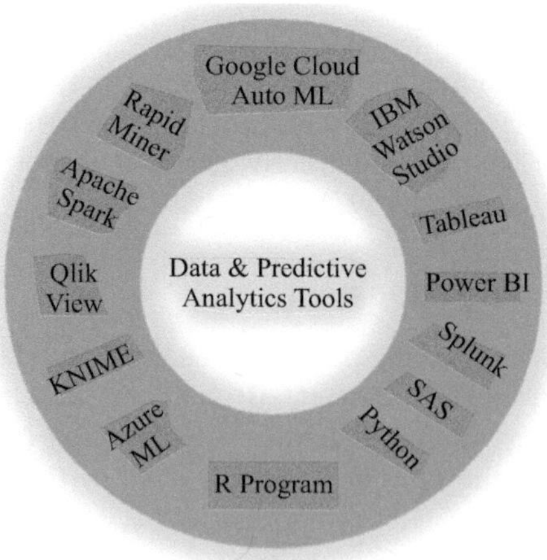

Fig. 3.3   Predictive analytics tools

Google Cloud AutoML

- AutoML is Google Cloud's automated machine learning tool.
- It allows users to build custom models without extensive knowledge of machine learning algorithms.
- The tool provides a user-friendly interface that can be easily accessed by anyone.
- AutoML provides excellent image, video, and text recognition capabilities.
- However, it has limited customization options compared to more advanced tools.

RapidMiner

- RapidMiner is an open-source predictive analytics tool that offers extensive functions of data mining functionalities.
- Its drag-and-drop interface enables users to build and deploy predictive models quickly.
- RapidMiner offers a comprehensive library of pre-built models and algorithms.
- It supports a vast array of data sources, making it a versatile choice.
- However, its lack of advanced visualizations and limited reporting features may be a disadvantage for some users.

Python with Scikit-learn

- Python, along with the Scikit-learn library, is a common choice for predictive analytics.
- It provides an extensive collection of machine learning algorithms, making it highly flexible.
- Python's vast community ensures a wealth of resources and support.
- The combination allows for deep customization and fine-tuning of models.
- However, working with Python and Scikit-learn requires coding skills and may be daunting for beginners.

There is a range of predictive analytics tools shown in Figure 3.3 each with its strengths and weaknesses. IBM Watson Studio and Microsoft Azure Machine Learning offer comprehensive platforms with advanced features. Google Cloud AutoML provides an accessible solution for users with limited technical expertise. RapidMiner caters to open-source enthusiasts, while Python with Scikit-learn allows for unparalleled customization. Choosing the appropriate tool depends on the particular requirements, budget limitations, and expertise of the users. Ultimately, selecting the right predictive analytics tool can greatly enhance a business's data-driven decision-making capabilities.

Predictive Analytics Algorithms

Predictive analytics algorithms are powerful tools used to study past and current data in order to create predictions about upcoming events or outcomes. These algorithms utilize a combination of statistical techniques, machine learning methods, and data mining approaches to discover patterns, trends, and associations within the entity. In Figure 3.4, we will explore various predictive analytics algorithms and their applications in different domains.

Linear Regression

The linear regression algorithm is a commonly used relationship between the variables and uses the least squares method to estimate the coefficients. Linear regression is commonly applied in sales forecasting, demand forecasting, and risk analysis.

Logistic Regression

Logistic regression is used to identify binary outcomes. It is widely used in areas such as fraud detection, credit counting, and customer churn prediction.

Decision Trees

Decision trees are popular algorithms that use a hierarchical structure to create predictions. They partition the data based on different attributes and can handle both definite and statistical variables.

Random Forests

Random forests are built on a random subset of features and generate a prediction. The ultimate prediction is determined by a majority vote or averaging of all the individual predictions. Random forests are robust against overfitting and are widely used in finance, marketing, and bioinformatics.

Support Vector Machines (SVM)

SVMs are effective in handling complex data with non-linear boundaries and are commonly used in image recognition, text classification, and bioinformatics.

Naive Bayes

Naive Bayes is a probabilistic algorithm based on Bayes' theorem and applied to spam filtering, document taxonomy and sentimentality analysis.

Neural Networks

Based on the human brain's biological neurons, neural network models are implemented and they consist of interconnected layers. They are used in image recognition, natural language processing, and recommendation systems.

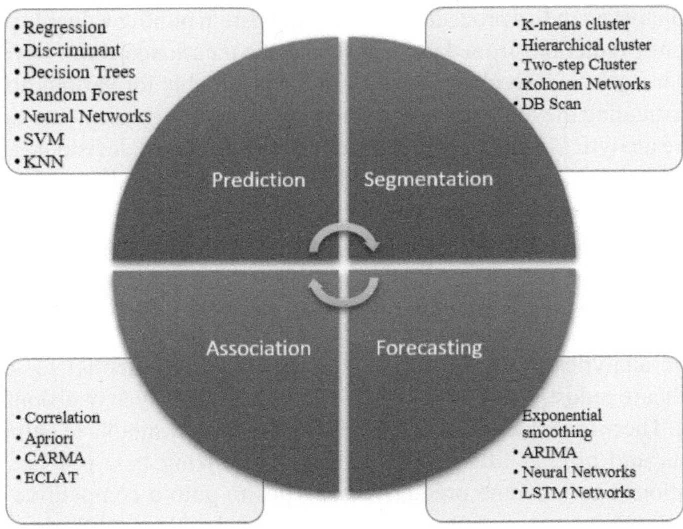

Fig. 3.4   Types of algorithms

Gradient Boosting

Gradient boosting is an ensemble learning technique that sequentially builds weak models, such as decision trees, and combines them to form a strong predictive model. Gradient boosting is widely used in Kaggle competitions, fraud detection, and personalized medicine.

Time Series Forecasting

Time series forecasting algorithms are specifically designed to predict future values based on past patterns and trends observed in time-ordered data. Popular algorithms for time series include ARIMA and RNNs. They are used in financial markets, energy demand forecasting, and inventory management.

Clustering

Clustering algorithms group similar instances together based on their attributes. They don't require any labeled data and are typically used for exploratory data analysis, customer segmentation, and anomaly detection.

Association Rules

Association rules are used to uncover patterns and associations in large datasets. They identify frequent item sets or groups of items that occur together. Association rules provide insights into customer behavior, market basket analysis, and product recommendations.

Predictive analytics procedures play a vital part in mining valuable perceptions and making predictions from data. The algorithms mentioned above have their own specific strengths and weaknesses, making them suitable for various applications. By understanding the fundamentals of these algorithms, organizations can leverage predictive analytics to gain a viable benefit, make informed decisions, and process optimization. Machine learning and artificial intelligence are able to propose a wide range of algorithms. However, the above-mentioned algorithms are specifically shown to predict chronic diseases as well as non-chronic diseases.

Disease Prediction Processing Model

Predictive analytics tools and methods offer immense potential for businesses, the healthcare industry and organizations to make data-driven decisions for future planning. There is a wide range of methods and models available to extract insights from data and predict future outcomes. By following best practice methods, organizations can leverage predictive analytics to gain a competitive edge. The optimization process of different phases shown in Figure 3.5, drives a better outcome model.

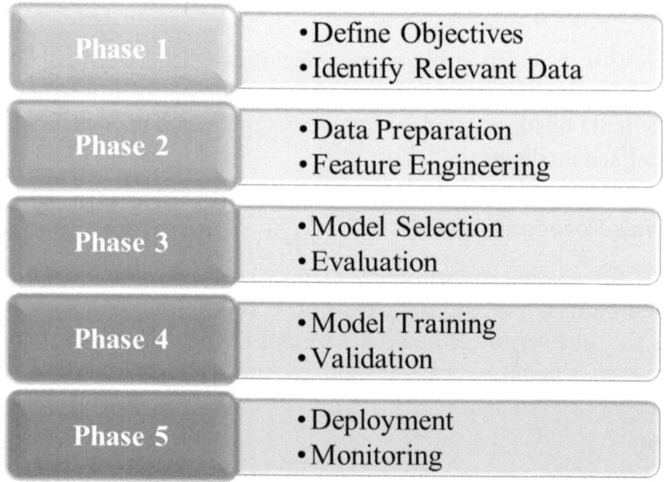

Fig. 3.5   Prediction process

The life cycle of predictive analytics in the realm of diagnosing diseases is a fascinating and dynamic process, involving data collection to modeling and implementation. This powerful tool has transformed healthcare by aiding in the early detection and accurate diagnosis of diseases, ultimately improving patient outcomes. Exploring the different phases of this life cycle and understanding how predictive analytics can be leveraged to enhance diagnostic capabilities is crucial.

Data Collection

The first step in the life cycle of predictive analytics is the collection of relevant data. This data could include patient medical records, laboratory test results, genetic information, lifestyle factors, and other pertinent details. With the advancement in electronic health records, data collection has become more streamlined, allowing for larger and more diverse datasets.

Data Preprocessing

Once the data is collected, it is crucial to preprocess and clean the data to eliminate inconsistencies and errors. This involves tasks such as handling missing data, removing outliers, and standardizing variables. The quality of the data greatly impacts the accuracy of the predictive models, so meticulous preprocessing is essential.

Feature Selection and Engineering

To develop effective predictive models, it is necessary to identify the most appropriate structures or entities from the dataset. Feature selection techniques help in reducing dimensionality, eliminating unnecessary variables, and retaining the most significant ones.

Model Development

Next comes the development of the predictive model. Various machine learning algorithms, such as decision trees, logistic regression, random forests, and neural networks, can be employed to build the model. Choosing the algorithm is based on the problem to be resolved, the available dataset, and the preferred level of accuracy. These models are trained using historical data, where the output (diagnosis) is known, and the input variables are used to predict future outcomes.

Model Evaluation and Validation

After designing a model, it needs to be verified for its performance. This is done by utilizing a portion of the dataset that was not used during the training phase. Metrics such as accuracy, precision, recall, and F1-score can be analyzed in order to evaluate the performance of the model. Validation techniques, such as cross-validation and bootstrapping, help ensure the model's generalizability and robustness.

Implementation and Deployment

Following rigorous assessment and validation, the predictive model is prepared for implementation. It can be integrated into the existing healthcare system to aid healthcare professionals in diagnosing diseases accurately. This may involve developing user-friendly interfaces or integrating the model into electronic health record systems. The implementation phase requires close collaboration between data scientists, healthcare providers, and IT professionals to ensure seamless integration into clinical workflows.

Monitoring and Maintenance

It is very important to constantly monitor its performance and keep informed about it periodically. Healthcare data is dynamic and subject to change, and therefore, the model needs to adapt to evolving trends and patterns. Feedback mechanisms and continuous evaluation aid recognize areas of improvement and accuracy.

Ethical Considerations

The ethical considerations regarding patient privacy, informed consent, bias in data, and interpretability of the model are critical aspects that need to be carefully addressed. Transparent communication with patients and healthcare professionals is essential to establish trust and ensure the responsible use of predictive analytics.

The life cycle of predictive analytics in diagnosing diseases is a multi-step process that encompasses data collection, preprocessing, feature selection, model development, evaluation, implementation, monitoring, and maintenance. It has the potential to revolutionize healthcare by providing accurate and timely diagnosis, leading to better treatment outcomes and improved patient care.

Optimization of Prediction Value

To maximize the effectiveness and reliability of prediction algorithms, several best practices should be followed to ensure accurate and reliable predictions.

Robust data governance

Establishing strong data governance frameworks ensures the collection, storage, and sharing of healthcare data in a secure and compliant manner. This comprises finding learned consent from individuals, confirming data privacy and security, and standing by relevant regulations and guidelines.

High-quality data collection

Collecting high-quality and comprehensive healthcare data is essential for perfect predictions. This includes ensuring standardization of data collection methods, reducing data biases, and considering data completeness and representativeness.

Model validation and recalibration

Prediction algorithms should undergo rigorous validation to assess their performance and reliability. Regular model recalibration is essential to account for changes in data distribution, population characteristics, and healthcare practices.

Transparency and interpretability

Ensuring transparency and interpretability is crucial for the adoption and trustworthiness of predictive models. Efforts should be made to make predictions and underlying algorithms explainable. This provides healthcare professionals and patients with clear insights into the factors influencing the predictions.

Collaborative approach

An alliance between medical practitioners, data scientists, policymakers, and patients is essential for the successful implementation of prediction algorithms. Such collaborations can help address the challenges related to data access, governance, and ethical considerations.

Still, experiments related to data obtainability, model interpretability, and ethical reflections must be addressed to confirm the effectiveness and answerable use of prediction algorithms in healthcare. By following best practices and fostering collaborations, we can harness the power of prediction algorithms to improve patient outcomes and transform healthcare delivery.

Future Advancements of Prediction Analytics in Health Care

Optimizing the use of predictive analytics in healthcare offers numerous benefits that can transform the industry. The future of prediction analytics in healthcare holds tremendous potential. Here are some possible advancements. It offers insights and predictions that can help improve patient outcomes, optimize resource allocation, and support informed decision-making. Advancements in technology, machine learning, and data analytics have laid the foundation for further developments in predictive analytics.

Real-Time Predictions

Real-time predictions hold immense potential in healthcare. With advancements in computing power and data processing capabilities, predictive models can now analyze vast amounts of data in real-time, leading to immediate insights and interventions. Real-time predictions can be particularly useful in emergency departments, enabling timely interventions and personalized decision-making based on up-to-date patient information.

Integration with Internet of Things (IoT)

The integration of predictive analytics with IoT devices and smart technology is a promising avenue for future development. Smart devices can provide continuous real-time data that can be analyzed using predictive analytics algorithms. This data can aid in early detection of health issues, monitoring chronic conditions, and facilitating personalized healthcare interventions.

Smart Wearable Devices Connectivity

The integration of prediction analytics with wearable devices can enable continuous monitoring of patient health. Real-time data from wearables such as heart rate monitors, glucose sensors, and activity trackers can be combined with prediction algorithms to provide personalized health insights.

Precision Medicine

By incorporating genomic data and other genetic markers into predictive models, healthcare professionals can predict disease susceptibility, treatment responses, and adverse drug reactions more accurately. This enables personalized treatment plans tailored to patients' unique genetic profiles, optimizing healthcare outcomes and reducing unnecessary treatments or adverse events.

Population Health Management

The future of predictive analytics in healthcare includes a focus on population health management. By analyzing large datasets and identifying trends, patterns, and risk factors within communities, healthcare organizations can develop targeted interventions to reduce disease burden and promote preventive care. Predictive models can help anticipate outbreaks, monitor population health indicators, and devise effective strategies to improve overall community well-being.

Enhanced Decision Support Systems

Predictive analytics can strengthen decision-making in healthcare by providing evidence-based insights and recommendations. Future advancements aim to develop more sophisticated decision support systems that enable clinicians to make more informed and precise decisions. By integrating patient data, medical knowledge, and predictive models, these systems can assist in diagnosis, treatment selection, and prognosis, thereby improving patient outcomes.

Predictive Analytics for Resource Allocation

Optimizing resource allocation is a critical aspect of healthcare management. Predictive analytics can support healthcare organizations in forecasting patient demand, supply needs, and resource allocation requirements. By analyzing past/ previous data and using predictive models, administrators can optimize the distribution of healthcare resources, such as hospital beds, staffing levels, and medical equipment, leading to improved operational efficiency and better patient care.

Collaboration and Data Sharing

The future of predictive analytics in healthcare calls for increased collaboration and data sharing among healthcare organizations. By pooling data from different sources, such as electronic health records, clinical trials, and research databases, predictive models can be refined and trained on larger, more diverse datasets. This can enhance the accuracy and generalizability of the simulations, prominent to more reliable predictions and perceptions.

Conclusion

Predictive analytics has become an indispensable tool in various industries, including healthcare. It involves utilizing past/previous data and statistical algorithms to sort predictions about future conclusions. The future of predictive analytics in healthcare holds immense potential for revolutionizing patient care, improving decision-making, and ensuring resource optimization. Real-time predictions, integration with IoT devices, precision medicine, population health management, enhanced decision support systems, and predictive analytics for resource allocation are just a few of the many exciting directions this field is evolving towards. However, addressing encounters associated with data privacy, quality, transparency, and ethical considerations is crucial to maximizing the benefits of predictive analytics and empowering healthcare professionals to make informed decisions for improved patient outcomes. The potential benefits of predictive analytics in healthcare are vast. By leveraging historical data and sophisticated algorithms, medical organizations can connect the influence of predictive analytics to improve patient care, increase working efficiency, and drive evidence-based decision-making. As technology continues to advance and healthcare data becomes more advanced and accessible, the role of predictive analytics in healthcare will only continue to grow, yielding significant advancements in patient care and population health.

References

Ahmed W., Fenton A., Hardey M. and Das R. 2022. Binge watching and the role of social media virality towards promoting Netflix's Squid Game. *IIM Kozhikode Society & Management Review*. 11(2):222–34.

Alam A. and Mohanty A. 2022. Predicting Students' Performance Employing Educational Data Mining Techniques, Machine Learning, and Learning Analytics. International Conference on Communication, Networks and Computing: (pp. 166–77). Cham: Springer Nature Switzerland.

Athiyarath S., Paul M. and Krishnaswamy S. 2020. A comparative study and analysis of time series forecasting techniques. *SN Computer Science*. 1(3):175.

Bharadiya J.P. 2023. Machine learning and AI in business intelligence: Trends and opportunities. *International Journal of Computer (IJC)*. 48(1):123–34.

Burger J., Isvoranu A.M., Lunansky G., Haslbeck J., Epskamp S. et al., 2022. Reporting standards for psychological network analyses in cross-sectional data. *Psychological Methods*.

Chatterjee A., Gerdes M.W. and Martinez S.G. 2020. Identification of risk factors associated with obesity and overweight—a machine learning overview. *Sensors*. 20(9):2734.

Feng M., Zheng J., Ren J., Hussain A., Li X. et al., 2019. Big data analytics and mining for effective visualization and trends forecasting of crime data. *IEEE Access*. 7:106111–23.

Fitzgerald R.C., Antoniou A.C., Fruk L. and Rosenfeld N. 2022. The future of early cancer detection. *Nature Medicine*. 28(4):666–77.

Hegde S.K. and Mundada M.R. 2022. Machine Learning-Based Approach for Predictive Analytics in Healthcare. In *Deep Learning Applications for Cyber-Physical Systems* (pp. 182–206). IGI Global.

Hossain M.E., Khan A., Moni M.A. and Uddin S. 2019. Use of electronic health data for disease prediction: A comprehensive literature review. *IEEE/ACM Transactions on Computational Biology and Bioinformatics*. 18(2):745–58.

Hoyos W., Aguilar J. and Toro M. 2023. PRV-FCM: An extension of fuzzy cognitive maps for prescriptive modeling. Expert Systems with Applications. 120729.

Ibrahim M.S. and Saber S. 2023. Machine Learning and Predictive Analytics: Advancing Disease Prevention in Healthcare. *Journal of Contemporary Healthcare Analytics*, 7(1), 53–71. Retrieved from https://publications.dlpress.org/index.php/jcha/article/view/16

Ishaq A., Sadiq S., Umer M., Ullah S., Mirjalili S. et al., 2021. Improving the prediction of heart failure patients' survival using SMOTE and effective data mining techniques. *IEEE access*. 9:39707–16.

Kang Y., Cai Z., Tan C.W., Huang Q. and Liu H. et al., 2020. Natural language processing (NLP) in management research: A literature review. *Journal of Management Analytics*. 7(2):139–72.

Khang A., Misra A., Gupta S.K. and Shah V. 2023. AI-Aided IoT Technologies and Applications for Smart Business and Production. CRC Press.

Kyrou I., Tsigos C., Mavrogianni C., Cardon G., Van Stappen V. et al., 2020. Sociodemographic and lifestyle-related risk factors for identifying vulnerable groups for type 2 diabetes: a narrative review with emphasis on data from Europe. *BMC Endocrine Disorders*. 20:1–3.

Lee A., Mavaddat N., Wilcox A.N., Cunningham A.P., Carver T. et al., 2019. BOADICEA: a comprehensive breast cancer risk prediction model incorporating genetic and nongenetic risk factors. *Genetics in Medicine*. 21(8):1708–18.

Lepenioti K., Bousdekis A., Apostolou D. and Mentzas G. 2020. Prescriptive analytics: Literature review and research challenges. *International Journal of Information Management*. 50:57–70.

Low D.M., Bentley K.H. and Ghosh S.S. 2020. Automated assessment of psychiatric disorders using speech: A systematic review. *Laryngoscope investigative otolaryngology*. 5(1):96–116.

Maheshwari S., Gautam P. and Jaggi C.K. 2021. Role of Big Data Analytics in supply chain management: current trends and future perspectives. *International Journal of Production Research*. 59(6):1875–1900.

Muniasamy A., Tabassam S., Hussain M. A., Sultana H., Muniasamy V. et al., 2020. Deep learning for predictive analytics in healthcare. In *The International Conference on Advanced Machine Learning Technologies and Applications (AMLTA2019) 4* (pp. 32–42). Springer International Publishing.

Nath P., Saha P., Middya A.I. and Roy S. 2021. Long-term time-series pollution forecast using statistical and deep learning methods. *Neural Computing and Applications*. 1–20.

Ngiam K.Y. and Khor W. 2019. Big data and machine learning algorithms for health-care delivery. *The Lancet Oncology*. 20(5):e262–73.

Ogbuke N.J., Yusuf Y.Y., Dharma K. and Mercangoz B.A. 2022. Big data supply chain analytics: ethical, privacy and security challenges posed to business, industries and society. *Production Planning & Control*. 33(2-3):123–37.

Park S., Xu Y., Jiang L., Chen Z. and Huang S. et al., 2020. Spatial structures of tourism destinations: A trajectory data mining approach leveraging mobile big data. *Annals of Tourism Research*. 84:102973.

Park Y.J., Fan S.K. and Hsu C.Y. 2020. A review on fault detection and process diagnostics in industrial processes. Processes. 8(9):1123.

Paulus J.K. and Kent D.M. 2020. Predictably unequal: understanding and addressing concerns that algorithmic clinical prediction may increase health disparities. *NPJ Digital Medicine*. 3(1):99.

Porsteinsson A.P., Isaacson R.S., Knox S., Sabbagh M.N. and Rubino I. et al., 2021. Diagnosis of early Alzheimer's disease: clinical practice in 2021. *The Journal of Prevention of Alzheimer's Disease*. 8:371–86.

Rajula H.S., Verlato G., Manchia M., Antonucci N. and Fanos V. et al., 2020. Comparison of conventional statistical methods with machine learning in medicine: diagnosis, drug development, and treatment. Medicina. 56(9):455.

Ravanelli M., Parcollet T., Plantinga P., Rouhe A., Cornell S. et al., 2021. SpeechBrain: A general-purpose speech toolkit. arXiv preprint arXiv:2106.04624.

Ray S., Das S.S., Mishra P. and Al Khatib A.M. 2021. Time series SARIMA modeling and forecasting of monthly rainfall and temperature in the South Asian countries. *Earth Systems and Environment.* 5:531–46.

Seyedan M. and Mafakheri F. 2020. Predictive big data analytics for supply chain demand forecasting: Methods, applications, and research opportunities. *Journal of Big Data.* 7(1):1–22.

Seyedan M. and Mafakheri F. 2020. Predictive big data analytics for supply chain demand forecasting: methods, applications, and research opportunities. *Journal of Big Data.* 7(1):1–22.

Shen Y., Yang W., Liu J. and Zhang Y. 2023. Minimally invasive approaches for the early detection of endometrial cancer. *Molecular cancer.* 22(1):53.

Sheng J., Amankwah-Amoah J., Khan Z. and Wang X. 2021. COVID-19 pandemic in the new era of big data analytics: Methodological innovations and future research directions. *British Journal of Management.* 32(4):1164–83.

Sheng J., Amankwah-Amoah J., Khan Z. and Wang X. 2021. COVID-19 pandemic in the new era of big data analytics: Methodological innovations and future research directions. *British Journal of Management.* 32(4):1164–83.

Souza P.C., Alessandri R., Barnoud J., Thallmair S., Faustino I. et al., 2021. Martini 3: a general purpose force field for coarse-grained molecular dynamics. *Nature Methods.* 18(4):382–88.

Tao D., Yang P. and Feng H. 2020. Utilization of text mining as a big data analysis tool for food science and nutrition. *Comprehensive reviews in food science and food safety.* 19(2):875–94.

Thapa C. and Camtepe S. 2021. Precision health data: Requirements, challenges and existing techniques for data security and privacy. Computers in biology and medicine. 129:104130.

Tursunbayeva A., Pagliari C., Di Lauro S. and Antonelli G. 2022. The ethics of people analytics: risks, opportunities and recommendations. *Personnel Review.* 51(3):900–21.

Zhao L. 2021. Event prediction in the big data era: A systematic survey. *ACM Computing Surveys (CSUR).* 54(5):1–37.

4

Machine Learning-Based Analysis for Detection of Pancreatic Adenocarcinoma Using Urinary Biomarkers

Shroddha Ghosh,[1] *Aleena Swetapadma,*[1*]
Satya Subham Nayak[1] and *Biswajit Sahoo*[1]

Pancreatic cancer poses a formidable challenge with its high fatality rate and asymptomatic progression until advanced stages. This study explores the potential of urinary biomarkers for spotting pancreatic cancer. The key biomarkers include creatinine, LYVE1, REG1B, and TFF1. It is collected from three patient groups such as healthy controls, non-cancerous pancreatic conditions and pancreatic ductal adenocarcinoma (PDAC). Age and sex factors are also considered as it is recognized as a contributor to pancreatic cancer. Differentiation between pancreatic cancer and non-cancerous conditions has been done by leveraging machine learning techniques, such as random forest (RF) method and light gradient boosting machine (LGBM) classifiers method. Results reveal promising insights into the diagnostic potential of urinary biomarkers, highlighting the significance of specific biomarkers in early pancreatic cancer identification. Furthermore, ensemble methods like bagging and AdaBoost are explored to enhance predictive performance, contributing valuable knowledge to the ongoing quest for an effective non-invasive diagnostic tool. The contribution of the work is that it can detect the PDAC with better accuracy than existing methods.

---

[1] School of Computer Engineering, KIIT Deemed to be University, Bhubaneswar, India

* Corresponding author: aleena.swetapadma@gmail.com

Introduction

Pancreatic cancer remains one of the most formidable challenges in oncology due to its notoriously high fatality rate. Early detection of pancreatic cancer is crucial as the disease often progresses silently until reaching advanced stages. In recent years, there has been a concerted effort to identify reliable diagnostic tools capable of detecting pancreatic cancer. Pancreatic cancer, particularly PDAC, presents a major global health concern due to its late-stage diagnosis and limited treatment options. PDAC is a devastating cancer with limited diagnostic options, emphasizing the urgent need for non-invasive and sensitive biomarkers. Notably, PDAC is known for its asymptomatic nature in the initial stages, making early diagnosis a formidable challenge.

This study delves into the promising realm of urinary biomarkers as potential indicators for pancreatic cancer detection. The study aimed at developing an accurate diagnostic test specifically for PDAC - pancreatic ductal adenocarcinoma. Key to this investigation are four urinary biomarkers. These biomarkers hold intrinsic value due to their potential associations with crucial physiological processes. Creatinine is included alongside LYVE1, a protein implicated in tumor metastasis. REG1B - regenerating family member 1 beta is known for its potential role in pancreas regeneration, while TFF1 - trefoil factor 1 constitutes another pivotal biomarker. The predictive task at hand involves discerning the diagnosis, specifically distinguishing between pancreatic cancer, non-cancerous pancreatic conditions, and individuals in good health. The primary objective is to develop a robust predictive model capable of identifying the presence of pancreatic cancer before formal diagnosis, thereby enhancing the prospects for timely intervention and improved patient outcomes.

Literature Survey

PDAC is a highly aggressive malignancy and detecting it is a very challenging task. The study about PDAC encompasses epidemiology, risk factors, diagnostic methods, treatment modalities, and ongoing research efforts. PDAC is a global health concern with a relatively low population-wide incidence but a disproportionately high mortality rate. Kriz et al., 2020 discussed that an estimated 140,116 new cases were reported in Europe alone, contributing to 132,134 deaths. Understanding the etiology of PDAC is complex. Established contributors include family history (3%-10% population attributable fraction), tobacco use, type-2 diabetes, obesity and blood group A/B (13%-19%). However, these factors alone do not fully account for the rising incidence, prompting further research into additional risk factors and gene-environment interactions. Efforts to establish screening programs for at-risk individuals, such as those with a strong family history or genetic susceptibility, face challenges in consensus regarding modalities and intervals. However, the lack of consensus on preferred modalities and the absence of robust data highlight the need for standardized screening approaches.

Liquid biopsies, focusing on biomarkers in body fluids, represent a promising avenue for early PDAC detection as suggested in (Wu et al., 2022). Current markers, such as CA 19-9, have limitations, prompting research into circulating tumor cells, circulating DNA (ctDNA), exosomes, and molecular analysis of pancreatic juice. Despite advancements, the field requires further validation in large-scale, multi-center trials to establish diagnostic accuracy. Curative therapy for PDAC often involves systemic chemotherapy but faces additional challenges in optimizing surgical outcomes and therapeutic sequences. Despite considerable advancements, the overall 5-year survival rate remains below 10%, underscoring the urgent need for innovative therapeutic strategies. The multifaceted nature of PDAC necessitates a collaborative, interdisciplinary approach to address the complex interplay of genetic, environmental, and clinical factors influencing the disease's progression and outcomes.

PDAC poses a significant challenge in early detection, contributing to its high mortality rate. A discussion in Karar et al., 2023 points out the potential of urinary biomarkers as potential diagnostic tools for PDAC. It focuses on urinary biomarkers, exploring their potential to revolutionize PDAC detection, prognosis, and monitoring. CA19-9, exhibits suboptimal sensitivity and specificity. The limitations of traditional biomarkers highlight the necessity for innovative approaches, leading to the exploration of urinary biomarkers. In the review by Acer et al., 2023 comparisons with traditional imaging modalities, such as CT and MRI, showcase the potential of urinary biomarkers as non-invasive alternatives. The integration of multiple diagnostic approaches could significantly enhance early detection rates. The evolving landscape of urinary biomarkers in PDAC necessitates continuous exploration. Urinary biomarkers offer a promising avenue for advancing PDAC diagnostics.

In Saraswathi H.S., and Rafi M. 2023, a literature review explores the recent advancements in utilizing machine learning (ML) techniques for the early detection of pancreatic cancer. A comprehensive analysis of studies, methodologies, and outcomes sheds light on the evolving landscape of ML applications in pancreatic cancer diagnosis. ML techniques have emerged as promising tools to enhance early detection, prognosis, and overall management of pancreatic cancer. ML algorithms help in the identification of subtle changes indicative of early-stage pancreatic cancer. They are used to analyze large-scale omics data to identify novel biomarkers associated with pancreatic cancer. The development of multiplex biomarker panels enhances the sensitivity and specificity of diagnostic tests.

ML algorithms applied to urine samples have shown promise in distinguishing pancreatic cancer patients from healthy controls as suggested in Ramachandra et al., 2023. It showcases the potential of ML-driven biomarker discoveries. Despite advancements, challenges such as data-set heterogeneity, limited sample sizes, and the need for standardized protocols remains. The robustness of machine learning models in pancreatic cancer detection can be enhanced through the integration of multi-modal data and collaborative efforts aimed at establishing large, diverse datasets. The integration of ML techniques in pancreatic cancer detection represents a paradigm shift, offering innovative solutions for early diagnosis that are crucial in the field of pancreatic cancer. This review emphasizes the diverse applications of

ML in imaging, biomarker discovery, and the analysis of urinary biomarker panels. It establishes a foundation for future research endeavors aimed at transforming pancreatic cancer management. In a specific study by Lee et al., 2021, both RF and the Cox proportional-hazards model were employed for predicting disease-free survival. The study suggests that artificial intelligence (AI) can be an important tool for analyzing patients. Another study by Liang et al. 2020 proposes a convolutional neural network (CNN)-based model. This literature review synthesizes current knowledge, emphasizing the potential of urinary biomarkers, the challenges faced in their implementation, and the collaborative efforts required for their successful integration into clinical practice. As research continues to unfold, urinary biomarkers stand poised as key players in the quest for early PDAC detection.

Techniques Used

The techniques employed in this study for PDAC detection primarily involve ML. However, the translation of ML models into clinical practice demands rigorous validation. Essential to this process are studies that assess the clinical applicability, scalability, and generalizability of ML-based diagnostic tools, fostering acceptance within the medical community. As the field progresses, future research should concentrate on refining existing ML algorithms, exploring novel data sources, and encouraging collaboration between computational scientists and clinicians. Prospective studies that integrate real-time data streams and facilitate continuous model refinement show promise for further enhancing early detection rates. Various ML techniques utilized in this work are detailed below.

Random Forest

The RF classifier utilized in this study is a random forest ensemble learning method. This algorithm constructs numerous decision trees during training, with each tree utilizing a subset of features and a random portion of the training data. The output is obtained using a voting mechanism, proving particularly beneficial for classification tasks. The mathematical foundation lies in the iterative construction of decision trees, each contributing to the model's predictive power. RF is renowned for its robustness, its ability to handle non-linear relationships, and its effectiveness in capturing intricate patterns in complex datasets. The architecture of the RF method is shown in Figure 4.1. In the context of cancer detection, such as in PDAC, RF excels in revealing nuanced relationships between input features and the target variable.

Light Gradient Boosting Machine

The LGBM classifier uses a gradient boosting framework. In contrast to traditional boosting methods, LGBM grows trees vertically in a leaf-wise manner, resulting in enhanced efficiency and speed. The mathematical underpinning involves minimizing the loss function by sequentially adding weak learners (trees). LGBM is

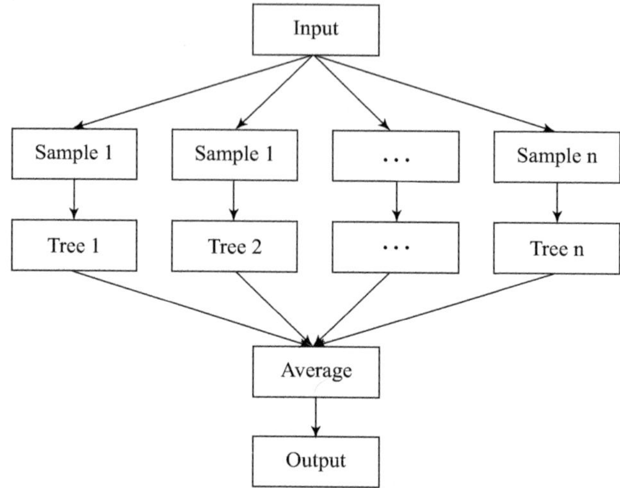

Fig. 4.1 Architecture of RF ensemble

particularly well-suited for scenarios with large datasets and a substantial number of features. In the context of cancer detection, especially in PDAC, LGBM's efficiency and ability to handle high-dimensional data make it an effective tool for capturing intricate patterns and making accurate predictions.

Bagging

It leverages the Bagging (Bootstrap Aggregating) meta-algorithm to enhance the stability and accuracy of the base classifier, which, in this case, is a random forest classifier. The bagging involves training with different bootstrap samples of the data-set and aggregating their predictions. This ensemble technique helps mitigate over-fitting and variance, resulting in a more robust and accurate model. In cancer detection applications, such as in PDAC, bagging proves advantageous by providing a more stable and reliable prediction mechanism.

Boosting

AdaBoost (Adaptive Boosting) is another ensemble learning method that sequentially enhances the performance of a weak classifier by assigning more weight to misclassified instances. The algorithm combines the predictions of weak learners through a weighted sum. In the context of cancer detection, AdaBoost can be beneficial for improving classification accuracy by focusing on challenging instances and emphasizing their importance in overall predictions.

Proposed Method

Pancreatic cancer, characterized by its high lethality, demands urgent attention to enhance early detection methods. The current diagnostic landscape faces significant challenges as the asymptomatic nature of pancreatic cancer often leads to late-stage diagnoses, resulting in a dismal prognosis. This research addresses the critical need for a robust and early detection tool for pancreatic cancer, specifically focusing on PDAC. The primary challenge lies in developing an accurate and reliable diagnostic model capable of distinguishing between three distinct groups. Leveraging urinary biomarkers such as creatinine, LYVE1, REG1B, and TFF1, collected from a diverse set of individuals, including healthy controls and those with non-cancerous pancreatic conditions, this study aims to unravel their potential in detecting the onset of PDAC. The ultimate goal is to contribute to the development of a non-invasive and efficient diagnostic tool. This research endeavors to increase survival rates for individuals diagnosed with pancreatic cancer. The proposed work consists of the following components as shown in Figure 4.2.

The steps of the proposed method are given below:

A. Data loading and processing: This component is responsible for loading and pre-processing the embroidery data.
B. Exploratory data analysis: This component is responsible for performing data analysis on the pre-processed data. This includes visualizing the data to identify patterns and trends and performing statistical analysis to identify relationships between variables.
C. Feature analysis and visualization: This component is responsible for identifying and extracting relevant features.
D. Model training: This component is responsible for training a classifier on the extracted features. The classifier will be used to predict the cluster labels for each embroidery sample.

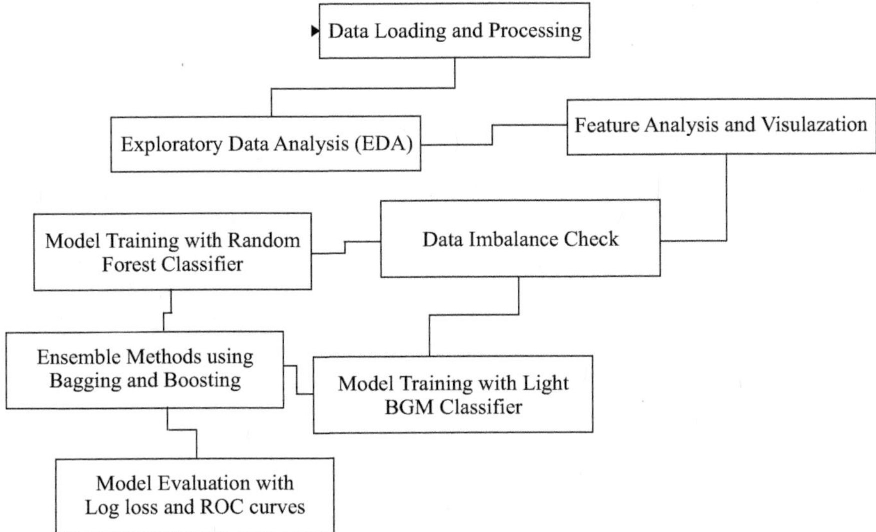

Fig. 4.2   Flowchart of the method

E. Data imbalance check: This component is responsible for checking the dataset for data imbalance. Data imbalance occurs when one class (e.g. the target class) is significantly more common than the other classes. If data imbalance is detected, appropriate techniques will be used to address it.

F. Ensemble methods (Bagging and AdaBoost): This component is responsible for training ensemble models using bagging and AdaBoost.

G. Model evaluation: This component is responsible for evaluating the performance using log loss and ROC scores. Log loss and ROC score are two metrics that are commonly used.

Dataset

This study explores the potential of urinary biomarkers for early detection, utilizing a dataset curated by Debernardi et al., 2020. The dataset includes crucial biomarkers such as plasma CA19-9, creatinine, LYVE1, REG1B, and TFF1, collected from three distinct patient groups: healthy controls, non-cancerous pancreatic conditions, and PDAC. Additionally, age and sex, recognized contributors to pancreatic cancer susceptibility, are taken into consideration.

Feature Importance

The dataset contains features such as plasma CA19-9, LYVEI, TFF1, REG18, age, sex and creatinine. To determine which features contribute more to the detection of PDAC, the following methods are employed.

Using Random Forest

Feature importance not only contributes to a deeper understanding of the underlying data dynamics but also enables strategic feature selection to optimize model performance. The theoretical underpinnings of RF variable importance emanate from the ensemble nature of the algorithm. In essence, RF aggregates decision trees, and during the training process, features that consistently contribute to reducing impurity across multiple trees are assigned higher importance scores. This amalgamation of diverse decision trees ensures robustness and adaptability to intricate data structures. Feature importance has been obtained using RF.

The image presented in Figure 4.3 illustrates the feature importance derived from an RF, reflecting the mean importance values across folds in a cross-validation procedure. The preeminent feature in this analysis is identified as plasma CA19-9, followed by LYVEI, TFF1, REG18, age, and creatinine. RF excels at computing feature importance by evaluating the extent to which each feature mitigates the impurity of the decision tree. The importance of a feature is gauged by its capacity to reduce impurity, where a higher reduction corresponds to greater importance. This intrinsic attribute of RF facilitates the discernment of influential features, thereby enhancing both model interpretability and predictive performance. The prominence of plasma CA19-9, LYVEI, TFF1, and REG18 in the feature importance ranking

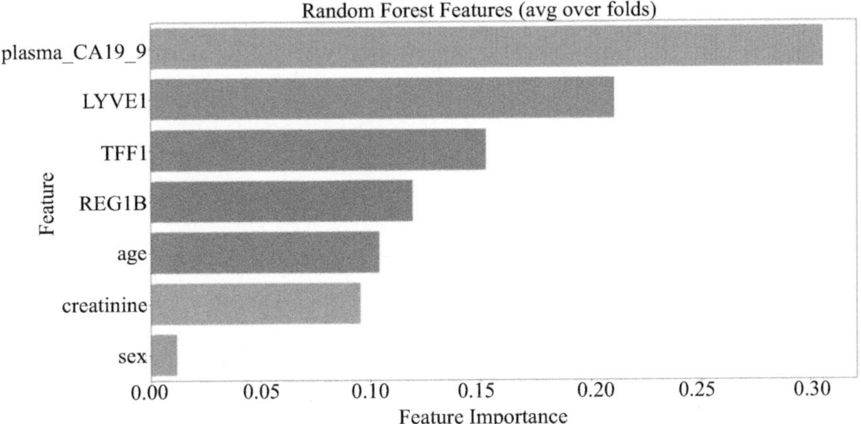

Fig. 4.3   Feature importance using random forest

underscores their pivotal roles in predicting the target variable. In conclusion, the feature importance analysis in the RF underscores the significance of plasma CA19-9, LYVEI, TFF1, and REG18 in predicting the target variable. This empirical investigation aligns with the broader theoretical framework of RF, wherein feature importance emerges as a critical facet for both interpretative insight and model refinement.

Using LGBM

LGBM is a gradient-boosting algorithm that shares conceptual roots with RF but distinguishes itself through enhanced computational efficiency. Notably, LGBM excels in accommodating diverse data types, including categorical variables, rendering it a versatile tool in predictive modeling. The theoretical underpinnings of variable importance in LGBM emanate from its ensemble learning structure. By iteratively constructing decision trees and emphasizing the importance of misclassified instances, LGBM refines its predictions and attributes higher importance to features that consistently contribute to accurate predictions across the ensemble.

The depicted image in Figure 4.4 encapsulates the feature importance output derived from an LGBM classifier, elucidating the significance of each feature within the model. The assigned importance scores are contingent upon the frequency with which a particular feature is employed to partition the data during the model's training. Higher importance scores denote a greater contribution of the feature to the predictive process. LYVEL emerges as the foremost feature in this analysis, followed by plasma CA19-9, creatinine, age, REG16, and TFFI. The prominence of these features signifies their substantive roles in informing and predicting the target variable within the model.

In the broader context of predictive modeling, the discernment of feature importance serves a dual purpose. Firstly, it affords a comprehensive understanding

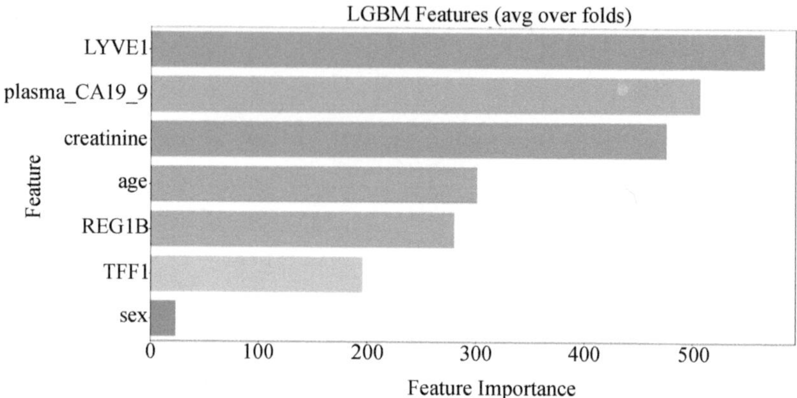

Fig. 4.4   Feature importance using LGBM

of the data dynamics, illuminating the features pivotal to predictive accuracy. Secondly, it facilitates strategic feature selection, thereby mitigating dimensionality and enhancing model interpretability. The ascendancy of LYVEL, plasma CA19-9, creatinine, and age as the foremost contributors to the target variable prediction underscores their informative prowess within the LGBM framework. This empirical revelation aligns seamlessly with the foundational tenets of LGBM, where feature importance assumes a central role in model interpretability and refinement.

Design of the proposed method

The perspective of this work extends beyond the creation of a predictive model; it focuses on designing an intelligent system that seamlessly aligns with the dataset, code, and overarching research goals. The core of system design revolves around harnessing the power of data science and machine learning. Python emerges as the language of choice, benefiting from its rich ecosystem of libraries such as NumPy, pandas, and sci-kit-learn. These tools serve as the sculptor's chisel, intricately carving patterns from the raw data. Understanding the resource demands of model training and evaluation is crucial. High-performance GPUs become accelerators, propelling the model through the intricate dance of feature extraction and classification. The urinary biomarkers, meticulously curated as input features for the detection of pancreatic cancer, undergo various trials. The final network structure is then selected for both classifiers. The module is thoroughly tested, and the results are discussed below.

Result

The proposed method has been validated, and its performance is discussed in this section. The performance metrics employed helps include accuracy and loss. Information loss, measured through cross-entropy, serves as a gauge of the alignment between model predictions and actual data, with lower values indicating heightened predictive accuracy.

Performance of LGBM

With Bagging

The evaluation of the LGBM classifier enhanced by bagging applied to the classification of PDAC, reveals commendable performance across key metrics, as detailed in Table 4.1. The model attains an accuracy of 91.01%, signifying its proficiency in correctly classifying PDAC cases within the test set. Precision and recall rate are 89.29% and 83.33% respectively. The F1 score stands at 86.21%, affirming the model's balanced performance crucial for robust PDAC classification. The Brier score loss, reflective of the model's probabilistic predictions, is 0.0899. Furthermore, the model exhibits an AUC for a bagging of 95.48%, highlighting its discriminative ability in distinguishing between PDAC and non-PDAC cases. The information loss, gauged through cross-entropy, is 0.2637, indicating the alignment of the model's predictions. Collectively, these metrics underscore the efficacy of the LGBM classifier with bagging as a promising tool for PDAC classification, demonstrating robust performance across diverse evaluative criteria.

Table 4.1   Performance of the LGBM method

Ensemble Type	Accuracy	Precision	Recall	F1-Score	ROC-AUC	Information Loss	Briar Score Loss
None	0.8764	0.88	0.73	0.8	0.9446	0.2823	0.1235
Bagging	0.9101	0.8285	0.83	0.86	0.9548	0.2637	0.08988
AdaBoost	0.8764	0.8275	0.8	0.81	0.9554	0.3748	0.12359

With Boosting

The evaluation of the LGBM classifier augmented by AdaBoost applied to the classification of PDAC, provides insights into its performance across pivotal metrics, as shown in Table 4.1. The model demonstrates an accuracy of 87.64%, reflecting its proficiency in correctly classifying PDAC cases within the test set. Precision, measured at 82.76%, underscores the model's ability to accurately identify instances classified as PDAC, thereby minimizing false positives. A recall rate of 80% signifies the model's capability to identify a considerable proportion of actual PDAC cases, mitigating false negatives. The F1-score, representing the harmonic mean of precision and recall, stands at 81.36%, indicating the model's balanced performance is essential for robust PDAC classification. The Brier score loss, indicative of the model's probabilistic predictions, is 0.1236. Additionally, the model exhibits an area under the curve (AUC) for AdaBoost of 95.54%, highlighting its discriminative ability in distinguishing between PDAC and non-PDAC cases. The information loss, gauged through cross-entropy, is 0.3748, signifying the alignment of the model's predictions with the actual data. These findings collectively characterize the LGBM Classifier with AdaBoost as a capable tool for PDAC classification, showcasing competitive performance across diverse evaluative criteria.

Performance of Random Forest Method

With Bagging

This research delves into a comprehensive examination of the RF with the bagging model's performance metrics in the context of PDAC classification utilizing urinary biomarkers, as outlined in Table 4.2. The evaluation encompasses key metrics, including accuracy (92.13%), highlighting the model's adeptness in correctly classifying PDAC cases within the test set. The ROC-AUC of 96.05% underscores the model's exceptional discriminatory prowess in distinguishing between PDAC and non-PDAC cases. Furthermore, a low information loss of 0.2596 signifies the model's predictions closely aligning with actual data, affirming the accuracy and reliability of its predictive capabilities. These findings collectively underscore the model's promising utility as a diagnostic tool for PDAC.

Table 4.2   Performance of the random forest method

Ensemble Type	Accuracy	Precision	Recall	F1-Score	ROC-AUC	Information Loss	Briar Score Loss
None	0.9101	0.8667	0.8667	0.8667	0.9613	0.2555	0.08988
Bagging	0.9213	0.9259	0.8333	0.8772	0.9605	0.2596	0.07865
AdaBoost	0.9101	0.8929	0.8333	0.8621	0.963	0.2491	0.08988

With Boosting

The model achieves an accuracy of 91.01%, denoting its efficacy in correctly classifying PDAC cases within the test set. Precision, measured at 89.29%, highlights the model's ability to accurately identify instances classified as PDAC, thereby minimizing false positives. The Brier score loss, indicative of the model's probabilistic predictions, is 0.0899. Additionally, the model exhibits an ROC-AUC of 96.30%, underscoring its exceptional discriminatory ability in distinguishing between PDAC and non-PDAC cases. The information loss, measured through cross-entropy, is low at 0.2491. These collective metrics substantiate the RF model with AdaBoost as a promising tool for PDAC classification, showcasing a strong performance across various evaluative criteria.

Discussion

The present study conducts a comparative analysis of two machine learning models, namely RF and LGBM, evaluating their performance metrics on a held-out test

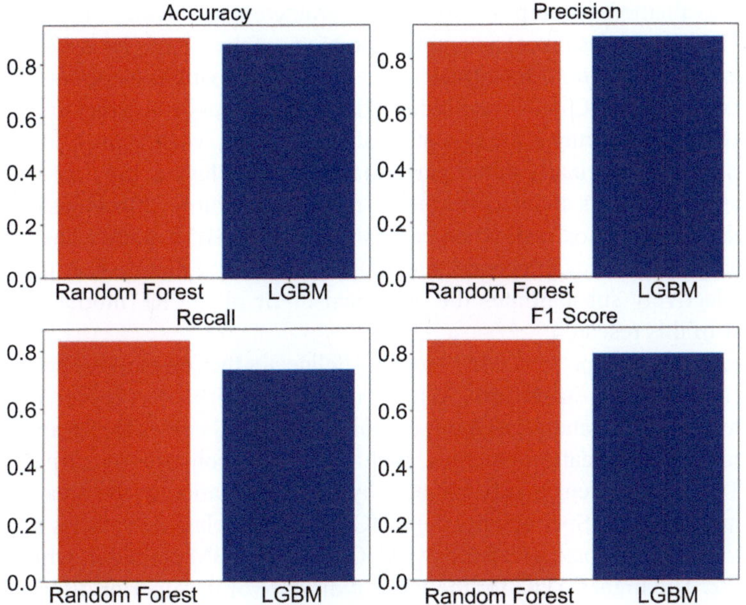

Fig. 4.5   Comparison of RF and LGBM

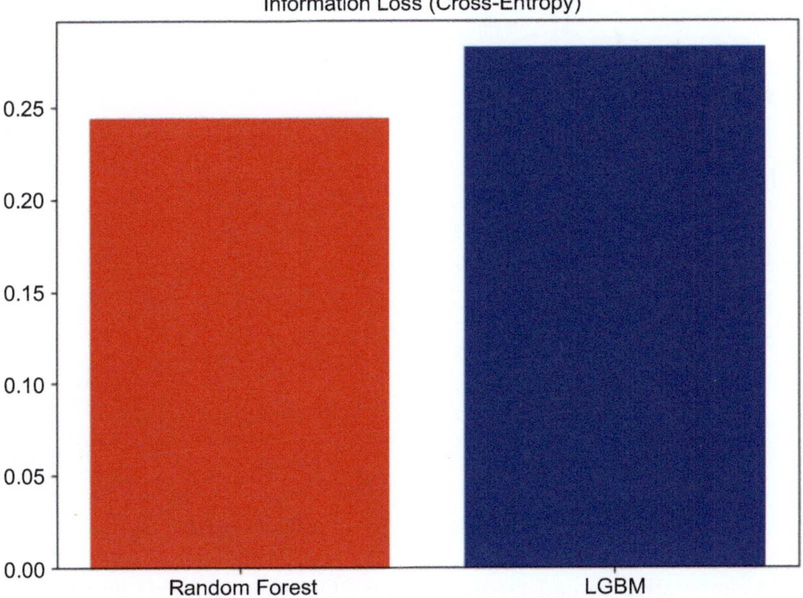

Fig. 4.6   Comparison of information loss

set. The evaluation encompasses different parameters as shown in Figure 4.5 and Figure 4.6 The results reveal a notable supremacy of the RF model across multiple performance indicators. Specifically, the RF model exhibits superior accuracy, precision, recall, ROC AUC, and reduced information loss compared to its LGBM counterpart. Noteworthy is the exception of the F1 score, wherein the LGBM model demonstrates a marginally better performance. In conclusion, the comprehensive assessment of metrics underscores the RF model as the more efficacious choice for the given classification task when compared to the LGBM model. The observed superiority in accuracy, precision, recall, ROC AUC, and diminished information loss collectively substantiates the empirical merit of the RF model within the purview of this research.

The ROC curve presented in Figure 4.7 delineates the comparative performance of RF and LGBM classifiers. Within the framework of receiver operating characteristic (ROC) analysis. Upon scrutinizing the ROC curves for RF and LGBM, a discernible stratification emerges, with the former consistently surpassing the latter. This discernment is substantiated by the computation of the area under the ROC curve (AUC). Specifically, the AUC for the RF classifier attains a value of 0.9664, surpassing the corresponding AUC for the LGBM classifier, which stands at 0.9412. The higher AUC for the RF is indicative of its superior discriminatory prowess in distinguishing between positive and negative instances compared to the LGBM classifier.

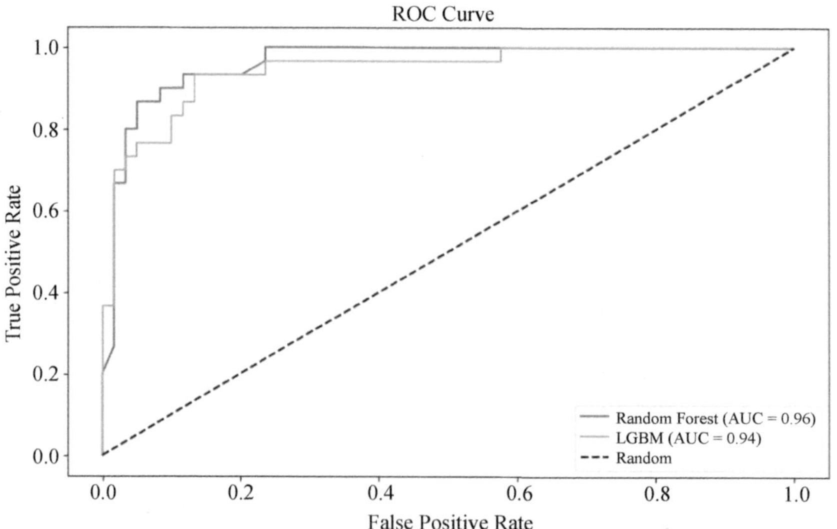

Fig. 4.7   Comparison of AUC of different methods

It is imperative to underscore that the ROC curve's x-axis and the y-axis represent the FPR and the TPR respectively. As a fundamental tenet of ROC analysis, an elevated curve corresponds to enhanced classifier performance. The idealized ROC curve manifests as a diagonal line from the bottom-left to the top-left corner. In this instance, the discernible elevation of the RF ROC curve above that of LGBM substantiates the former's superior discriminating capacity. In summation, the empirical evidence encapsulated within the ROC analysis posits the RF classifier as exhibiting heightened proficiency compared to its LGBM counterpart. The quantified AUC differential and the visually elevated ROC curve collectively affirm the superior performance of the RF classifier in the discrimination of positive and negative instances within the purview of the examined data-set.

Conclusion

In this study, PDAC detection has been accomplished using machine learning and biomarkers, with the RF method proving more accurate than the LGBM method. Prospective research endeavors are poised to concentrate on meticulous model refinement through nuanced feature engineering, potentially exploring additional urinary biomarkers and incorporating advanced data pre-processing techniques to augment the predictive efficacy of the models. Additionally, the integration of urinary biomarker data with pertinent clinical information remains an avenue for comprehensive diagnostic insights, where the inclusion of patient demographics, medical history, and imaging data could contribute to a more holistic understanding of PDAC. The future utility of the models extends towards real-time applications within clinical settings, facilitating timely decision-making and improving patient outcomes. The seamless integration of these models into healthcare systems is anticipated to play a pivotal role in early detection and diagnosis. Moreover, the models warrant further validation through cross-validation and external assessments, especially on diverse datasets from varying populations or clinical contexts, to ensure robust generalizability. Future research efforts are mandated to focus on the development of strategies that address biases within the data, ensuring equitable and fair model predictions. The future trajectory of the developed models for PDAC classification, particularly emphasizing the RF model in both its bagging and boosting configurations, holds substantial promise for further refinement and expansion in clinical applications. In summation, the future trajectory of the developed PDAC classification models underscores a comprehensive approach encompassing continual improvement, seamless integration into clinical practices, and the adept navigation of emerging challenges to fortify the nexus between data science and medical expertise for optimized patient care and outcomes.

References

Acer I., Bulucu F.O., Icer S. and Latifoglu F. 2023. Early diagnosis of pancreatic cancer by machine learning methods using urine biomarker combinations, *Turkish Journal of Electrical Engineering and Computer Sciences*, 31(1), 8.

Debernardi S., Brien H., Algahmdi A.S., Malats N., Stewart G.D. et al., 2020. A combination of urinary biomarker panel and PancRISK score for earlier detection of pancreatic cancer: A case- control study, *PLoS Med.*, 7(12), e1003489.

Kaggle dataset: & quot; Urinary Biomarkers for Pancreatic Cancer", https://www.kaggle.com/datasets/johnjdavisiv/urinary-biomarkers-for-pancreatic-cancer

Karar M.E., El-Fishawy N. and Radad M. 2023. Automated classification of urine biomarkers to diagnose pancreatic cancer using 1-D convolutional neural networks. *J Biol Eng.*, 17(1), 28.

Kriz D., Ansari D. and Andersson R. 2020. Potential biomarkers for early detection of pancreatic ductal adenocarcinoma. *Clin Transl Oncol.*, 22(12), 2170–74.

Lee K.S., Jang J.Y., Yu Y.D., Heo J.S., Han H.S. et al., 2021. Usefulness of artificial intelligence for predicting recurrence following surgery for pancreatic cancer: Retrospective cohort study. *International Journal of Surgery*, 93, 106050.

Liang Y., Schott D., Zhang Y., Wang Z., Nasief H. et al., 2020. Auto-segmentation of a pancreatic tumor in multi-parametric MRI using deep convolutional neural networks. *Radiother Oncol.*, 145, 193–200.

Ramachandra H.V., Chavan P., Ali A. and Ramaprasad H.C. 2023. Ensemble Machine Learning Techniques for Pancreatic Cancer Detection, International Conference on Applied Intelligence and Sustainable Computing, India, 1-5.

Saraswathi H.S. and Rafi M. 2023. Promising urinary biomarkers to predict Pancreatic Ductal Adenocarcinoma using machine learning techniques. *Eur. Chem. Bull.*, 12 (8).

Wu H., Ou S., Zhang H., Huang R., Yu S. et al., 2022. Advances in biomarkers and techniques for pancreatic cancer diagnosis. *Cancer Cell Int*, 22, 220.

5

Gland Segmentation in Colon Histology Images Using Deep Learning Method

Aditi Sharma,[1] *Poojasri Inagala,*[1] *Jayesh Gangrade*[1*] and *Hemlata Parmar*[1]

The high death rates and incidences of colorectal cancer make it a serious worldwide health problem. Colorectal cancer is a malignancy that is prevalent and concerning. There are various factors that may add to the formation of this disease. These factors include genetics, family history, lifestyle choices, and environmental conditions. Hence it is essential that solutions for effective diagnosis and treatment be researched and developed. This research proposed the U-Net model architecture, a deep-learning technique to determine glandular structures in histological images of the colon. Segmentation of images is carried out using the U-Net architecture, a framework of deep learning, notably in the field of medicine. In recent years, it has shown amazing effectiveness in the identification of abnormalities, such as tumors, in medical images. We utilized the Warwick-QU dataset, a valuable resource provided as part of the GlaS challenge. This dataset comprises images of slides that were subjected to hematoxylin and eosin (H&E) staining, expertly annotated by professionals with expertise in the medical field. Leveraging this dataset, we trained the U-Net model to accurately segment glandular structures and malignant tissues in colon histology images.

[1] Department of Artificial Intelligence, School of Computer Science & Engineering, Manipal University, Jaipur, India.

* Corresponding author: jayesh.gangrade@jaipur.manipal.edu

Introduction

The colon, the longest segment of the large intestine, assumes a pivotal role in the digestive process. It serves as the recipient of partially digested food, facilitates its further processing, and streamlines the absorption of vital nutrients. Following the absorption phase, the colon directs waste materials towards the rectum for eventual excretion (Colorectal Cancer Statistics | How Common Is Colorectal Cancer? 2023). Nevertheless, the emergence of malignancies in the colon can be attributed to uncontrolled and aberrant cellular division, which leads to irregular cell growth. This oncogenic transformation is primarily driven by genomic alterations, often referred to as "gene mutations," and serves as a catalyst for the disease's progression. These mutations disrupt the natural cell life cycle by enabling affected cells evade apoptosis, unlike their healthy counterparts (Colorectal Cancer Statistics | How Common Is Colorectal Cancer? 2023). Colorectal cancer can affect individuals at various stages of life, although it predominantly afflicts adults (Colorectal Cancer Statistics | How Common Is Colorectal Cancer? 2023). Over time, clusters of cells congregate to form polyps, small growths within the colon. These polyps are of concern due to their typically asymptomatic nature, underscoring the necessity for regular screening as a preventive measure and for early detection to facilitate more effective treatment plans (Colorectal Cancer Statistics | How Common Is Colorectal Cancer? 2023, Colorectal Cancer – Statistics 2023).

Consequently, there exists a pressing demand for comprehensive research and meticulous analysis within this domain. The delineation and precise segmentation of glandular structures in histopathological images constitute a pivotal aspect of early disease detection, the assessment of its severity, and the formulation of an appropriate treatment strategy (Colorectal Cancer Statistics | How Common Is Colorectal Cancer? 2023). Gland segmentation denotes the precise identification of potentially malignant structures embedded within the histopathological images of patients, serving as a critical endeavor in the field of medical diagnostics (Colorectal Cancer Statistics | How Common Is Colorectal Cancer? 2023).

These structures undergo meticulous scrutiny, with an emphasis on factors such as spatial arrangements, dimensions, and morphology, which collectively contribute to the assessment of the presence or absence of polyps (Sirinukunwattana et al., 2017). In this study, a method based on deep learning is introduced for the precise segmentation of glandular structures within colon histology images, employing the U-Net model architecture. This approach has been rigorously tested and trained using the dataset from Warwick-QU as part of the GlaS challenge (Gland segmentation in Colon Histology Images). The dataset comprises a diverse array of samples extracted from various patients, comprising of images of Slides that were subjected to hematoxylin and eosin (H&E) staining, along with corresponding ground truth annotations meticulously provided by professionals in the field of medicine and pathology (Sirinukunwattana et al., 2017). The central focus of this study lies in evaluating the efficacy of the UNet architecture in image segmentation, with particular attention to its feature-capturing capabilities. This research is driven by the motivation to leverage deep learning techniques via the UNet model architecture to perform image segmentation, with the primary goal of identifying malignant tissues. The evaluation of the performance of the model was done by various parameters such as the Dice coefficient, Intersection over Union (IOU), model performance, number of training epochs, and loss function, specifically based on the Dice coefficient.

Contributions

- Applying deep learning in the field of Medical Sciences for analysis of colorectal cancer with the help of images.
- Providing an introduction to gland segmentation in colon histology using the UNet method.
- Training the model using the Warwick-QU dataset and then evaluating its performance using various performance metrics like the Intersection Over Union and Dice coefficient for an In-depth assessment.
- Laying the foundation for future research in gland segmentation techniques and demonstrating the potential of CNN-based UNet in the field of Medical Sciences for the detection of colorectal cancer.

Literature Review

In 2022, Tharwat et al. conducted research using deep learning and image analysis from medicine and histology to study the early identification and treatment of colon cancer. They took into consideration some characteristics like symptoms, grades and imaging methods and aimed to enhance the automated diagnostic techniques. The study examined the merits and demerits of machine learning and deep learning techniques by using datasets such as the colorectal histology images (CCOHIS). The discussion here was about various algorithms, including Support Vector Machines, Random Forests, and K-nearest neighbors, with feature extraction from histology images strengthening diagnostic processes, and deep-learning techniques like Convolutional Neural Networks were reviewed to identify patterns that may be linked to cancer growth stages. All these tools may aid in the early detection and diagnosis of disease and hence with early treatment, the death rates can be lowered. The focus needed to be on the importance of more research in the field and to perform a future comparative examination of deep learning and machine learning methods. However, it failed to offer a singular dataset for training and testing the model thoroughly, doesn't have sufficient methods for testing, and lacks a thorough analysis of the approaches applied and the limitations of methods in use. Our study, in collaboration with the cited paper, highlights the importance of detection of cancer at the early stages. Extending the paper's analysis of various machine-learning approaches, our research explores the segmentation of glands using the UNet model. This helps to contribute to the objectives of the cited work and to provide insightful research in the field (Tharwat et al., 2022).

In 2019, Rezai et al. conducted research that focuses on properly segmenting glands in histological images, which is vital for the identification of disease. To improve gland segmentation precision and utility, the researchers used a mixed approach that is a combination of deep neural networks with manually created features. The approach employed a one-of-a-kind modification of the LinkNet architecture as well as custom features, most notably the invariant local binary pattern (LBP). The study focused on the usage of red and hematoxylin channels as input, as well as the post-processing methods which include the Otsu method and morphological processes, for the improvement in the quality of glandular segmentation. Experiments were carried out on the Warwick-QU dataset, and the system showed that it could distinguish between glands as well as identify cancerous areas. However, it failed to include the limitations of the suggested approach and failed to address the computational requirements and the efficiency of the proposed system. These are some of the critical factors for implementation in the real world. Our study, in collaboration with the cited paper, focuses on a common goal of the detecting diseases using segmentation techniques – especially through deep neural networks. Our study uses the UNet Model and evaluates the performance on various metrics like the Dice coefficient and IOU, which is in line with the focus of the cited paper on thorough model testing (Rezaei et al., 2019).

In 2023, Nasir et al. conducted research that provides a comprehensive assessment of techniques based on artificial intelligence for the segmentation of glands and nuclei in histology images, and the analysis of 126 AI-based methods in this field. It evaluated methods that exist already, revealing flaws and paving the way for future research. The research included input from accessible datasets, as well as classic handmade feature extraction approaches including intensity-based thresholding and morphological procedures, as well as deep learning-based neural network techniques. It considered the performance of R-CNN and its variations sufficient but in histopathological tasks, they have limitations. The investigation was necessary due to two challenges namely data scarcity and color inconsistency to improve segmentation accuracy. Future promise might be seen in techniques such as FCN-based Atrous spatial pyramid pooling and Encoder-Decoder U-Nets. Deep CNN integration with post-processing techniques and symmetrical network designs were also interesting. Whereas, addressing staining variances and limited training data in deep learning models, was critical. Accurate segmentation of complex structures remained a major challenge. It, however, failed to provide the developer validation of the algorithm resulting in challenges with potential bias, low repeatability, and limited applicability making it difficult to resolve important issues. The cited paper examined prior approaches and highlights the limitations that guide our use of the UNet model for the segmentation of glands. Based on the groundwork set by the cited paper, our work addresses shared problems such as the scarcity of training data and staining variability to depict how advancement in this field can contribute to early detection and diagnosis of colorectal cancer (Nasir et al., 2023).

In 2021, Dabass et al. conducted research that introduces a deep learning technique called The Attention-Guided Deep Atrous-Residual U-Net. This technique was developed particularly with the intent of gland segmentation in colon histopathology images. It employed unique, multi-tiered feature representations with Atrous-Residual units to handle diminishing gradients. The attention units were used to extract accurate gland-specific characteristics, resulting in the improvement of semantic feature concatenation. Resolution degradation and multi-scale characteristics were addressed by Atrous units. Model performance was assessed using two datasets: the GlaS challenge, CRAG, and a private hospital dataset (HosC). To help in improving the model's generalization capability, the model utilized various strategies like "Multiple data augmentation and stain normalization". Various performance indicators were used to check the model's competitiveness and advantages over earlier methodologies. They were—the F1-score, Object-Dice Index, and Object-Hausdorff Distance. With the addition of atrous-residual units, attention units, and transitional atrous units to the architecture, the model's ability to capture small details and correctly segment glands were enhanced. By addressing concerns such as data unpredictability, overfitting, and resolution deterioration, this significant achievement had huge potential for colon cancer diagnosis. Future studies could broaden its application to histopathological images of other organs, improving its clinical utility. The failure to address the limitations of the proposed method could make the evaluation of robustness and application of the method more difficult. The cited paper aligns with our focus on the application of UNet architecture for better accuracy by proposing advanced techniques for image segmentation in colon histopathology images. Enhancements to our model are guided by the shared use of performance metrics like the Dice coefficient and insights from Attention and Atrous-Residual units (Dabass et al., 2021).

A 2020 research conducted by Kosov et al. focuses on accurately representing the mucous glands in histological images provided by the dataset. Upon applying this method, gland shapes were used for generating probabilistic representations of glandular boundaries, and the findings obtained by the segmentation of images were enhanced by using a convolutional neural network (CNN). When it came to automated histological gland segmentation, the technique was especially good at successfully dividing adjacent glands. Using real histological pictures of colon tissue from the Warwick-QU dataset, the study assessed the suggested method. The study highlighted how important accurate gland segmentation was to get reliable morphological data. This was essential in developing efficient algorithms for diagnosis and guaranteeing timely medical intervention. The suggested method considered the geometric properties of histological glandular structures, which resulted in the development of a probability map. The approach is rooted exclusively in the mathematical basis of image processing. Methods that incorporate traditional image processing methods, machine learning approaches at one or multiple stages, are completely dependent on the implementation of neural network models. It failed to address the computational efficiency of the proposed approach which holds significance for practical real-time application implementation. Moreover, it doesn't address certain challenges such as the impact of segmentation of glands with varying shapes and sizes on accuracy and fails to discuss the robustness of the proposed method to frequently arising problems like changes in image quality and straining. The cited paper aligns with our research by discussing gland segmentation in histopathological images of colorectal cancer. The shared use of the Warwick-QU dataset and various performance metrics, such as IOU and the Dice coefficient helps to strengthen this alignment and guide our findings (Kosov et al., 2020).

In a research conducted in 2021, Hamida et al., the application of deep learning (DL)-based architectures was examined, for the identification and categorization of areas associated with colon cancer in histopathology images. Modern convolutional neural networks (CNNs), such as AlexNet, VGG, ResNet, DenseNet, and Inception, were reviewed in depth in this paper. To determine these models' efficacy in this situation, comparisons were made between them. To circumvent the constraints caused by the lack of large Whole Slide Image (WSI) datasets, transfer learning methods were utilized. This entails using ImageNet, a sizable computer imaging dataset, for training networks with the objective of extracting a variety of learned features. Numerous datasets, such as the AI COLO colon cancer dataset, CRC-5000, nct-crc-he-100k, were utilized with combined datasets to rigorously evaluate DL models. The models reached surprisingly high accuracy rates, which was impressive. It failed to provide basic characteristics of the dataset, such as sample size which limited the scope of the findings. Also, for the evaluation of performance, only accuracy was considered and other important metrics like precision, recall, and F1 score were ignored which limited the evaluation of the model's efficiency. The cited paper aligns with our research on the topic of the application of deep learning for the treatment of colorectal cancer. Both works highlight the efficiency of CNNs in the identification of irregularities within the tissues and cells of the colon with a mutual goal of promoting the detection and diagnosis of colorectal cancer using new and innovative technologies (Hamida et al., 2021).

In their 2022 research in 2022, Davri et al., 2022 conducted an in-depth examination of the current state of using deep learning algorithms, a particular type of sophisticated technology in the analysis of colorectal cancer (CRC) images. The focus primarily lay on using these algorithms to help with CRC diagnosis as well as prognosis in histopathological circumstances. The diagnosis of CRC could be done in a better way with the help of Deep Learning algorithms, forecasting vital molecular characteristics, and recognizing microsatellite instability. In addition, these algorithms had the ability to assess elements of the tumor microenvironment and identified particular histological characteristics linked to metastasis and prognosis. This study focused on the increasing need for trustworthy machine-assisted techniques in pathology diagnosis, mainly because of the increasing volume of diagnostic cases and the unpredictability of biomarker evaluation. Utilizing deep learning techniques, researchers wanted to improve precision. It failed to provide information about the characteristics of included studies in the systematic review which hampers the applicability of results. Additionally, it was difficult to fully comprehend the results because of the lack of addressing limitations of the model and potential biases. The cited paper underlined the use of deep learning techniques, which aligned with our work based on the UNet model. Both works highlight the importance of accurate analysis and aim to improve the detection and diagnosis of CRC using advanced technologies primarily deep learning (Davri et al., 2022).

In a research in 2017, Hamad et al. researched the incorporation of deep learning techniques, such as a CNN, to navigate the difficult task of dividing nuclei, cells, and tissues in colon cancer and the histology of slides. This deep learning method effectively segregated colon cancer nuclei into four groups: miscellaneous, fibroblast, inflammatory, and epithelial. The CNN model, which had six layers—convolution, subsampling, fully linked, and output layer, managed the difficulties caused by differences in cell morphologies and staining techniques well. Using a sizable dataset of photos of colon cancer nuclei, the authors analyzed the system's effectiveness using a weighted average F1 score. Their approach worked extremely well compared to previous approaches, demonstrating its effectiveness in medical analysis. This study enlightened how deep learning can implement complex structural properties. It failed to provide important details regarding the dataset such as the size. This may potentially restrict the applicability of the model and it also ignores the possibility of potential biases or limitations in ground truth nucleus locations which might impact the accuracy of the results. The cited paper aligns with our research which focuses on the application of deep learning, especially CNNs for an accurate and improved diagnosis of colorectal cancer. Both works underline the significance of precise segmentation of glands which can contribute towards an improved diagnosis in the medical field (Hamad et al., 2017).

Methodology

Convolutional Neural Networks (CNNs) is a type of deep learning technique that has become a more powerful tool for medical image processing because of recent developments in the field (Hamida et al., 2021). CNNs, or Convolutional Neural Networks, are specialized in processing and interpreting visual data, demonstrating exceptional accuracy in identifying structures and patterns within medical images. Moreover, they possess the capability to learn and extract intricate features from complex medical images, further enhancing their utility in the field (Kainz et al., 2017). The application of CNNs and deep learning techniques in medical science, particularly in the context of colon gland segmentation, holds the potential to achieve precise glandular segmentation, thereby facilitating accurate results and, crucially, early detection not only in cases of colon cancer but also in the context of diseases affecting other vital organs.

U-Net Architecture

The field of machine learning includes deep learning, which employs artificial neural networks to gather and analyze intricate features from large, complicated data (Zhang. 2021). The UNet model architecture, a specific type of CNN, is predominantly employed for image segmentation within the medical field, particularly for biomedical images (Maynard-Reid. 2023). The UNet architecture, which comprises the contracting path and the expanding path, efficiently employs skip connections to establish links between the two paths (Khazaee et al., 2023).

The segment known as the contracting path, often referred to as the encoder, plays a crucial role in the initial stages of image transformation. It involves a series of systematic steps commencing with the input image. These steps encompass the application of convolutional layers, functioning akin to filters, to analyze the image by scanning it with small receptive fields for the extraction of specific features (K.B. 2021; Kirouane. 2022; O'Sullivan. 2023; Adaloglou. 2021). Following each convolutional layer, a max-pooling operation is implemented to reduce both the spatial properties of the image. and concurrently augment the feature maps or the number of channels. The total number of channels doubles with every iteration of the process, which is repeated several times. (K.B. 2021; Kirouane. 2022; O'Sullivan, 2023; Adaloglou. 2021).

The repetition of operations in the contracting path, commonly referred to as the encoder, serves the pivotal purpose of capturing increasingly intricate and complex patterns within the image (Zhang. 2021; O'Sullivan. 2023). As this process culminates, it arrives at a bottleneck layer, strategically positioned to encapsulate the most critical features present in the input image (Zhang. 2021; O'Sullivan. 2023). On the other hand, the expanding path, also known as the decoder, assumes the role of generating the final segmentation map. It accomplishes this by upsampling the features from the bottleneck layer and integrating them with the features obtained from the contracting path through the utilization of skip connections. To achieve upsampling, transposed 2D convolutional layers are employed (Zhang. 2021; O'Sullivan. 2023). The introduction of skip connections plays a pivotal role in retaining specific details in the image, facilitating the delineation and segmentation of distinct parts of the image (GeeksforGeeks. 2023) Consequently, the output takes the form of a segmentation map, preserving the spatial dimensions akin to those of the original input image, where each pixel represents a class label (Zhang 2021; GeeksforGeeks. 2023).

Dataset

The dataset utilized in this study originates from the Warwick-QU dataset, which is a constituent of the GlaS (Gland segmentation in Colon Histology Images challenge). This particular dataset consists of 165 images, each formatted in BMP, and sourced from 16 histological sections that were subjected to hematoxylin and eosin (H&E) staining. These sections pertain to colorectal adenocarcinoma cases categorized as stage T3 or T4. Notably, the images represent distinct patient samples. Each image within this dataset is accompanied by a single ground truth object corresponding to a label (Sirinukunwattana et al., 2015, 2017).

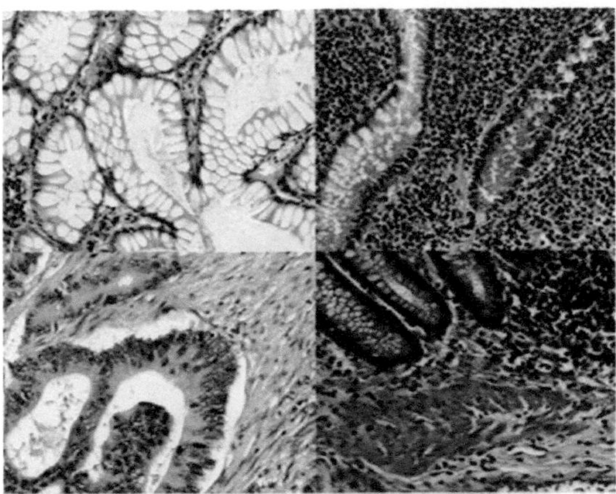

Fig. 5.1   Histopathological images from dataset

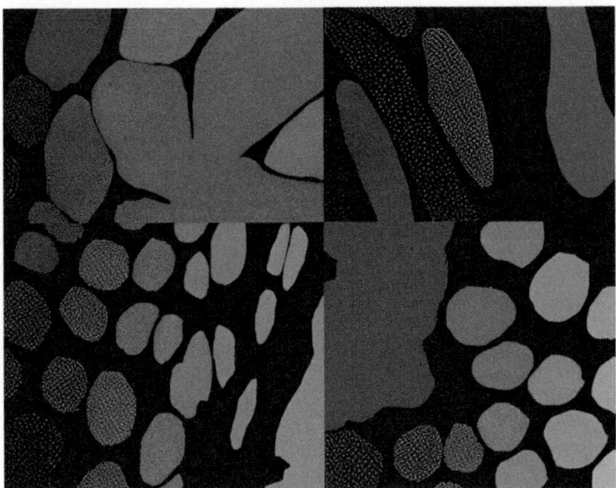

Fig. 5.2   Masks for these images from dataset

Methodology

Our comprehensive methodology for developing a medical image segmentation model centers around ten well-defined steps, driven by the renowned U-Net architecture and underpinned by the dataset from Warwick-QU which was taken from the GlaS challenge.

In the initial phases, we carefully select the U-Net model, well-regarded for its aptness in medical image segmentation. This is followed by rigorous data preprocessing and loading, which standardizes image and mask dimensions to 256×256 pixels and normalizes pixel values within [0, 1]. In the third step, some performance metrics to assess the model's performance have been used like the

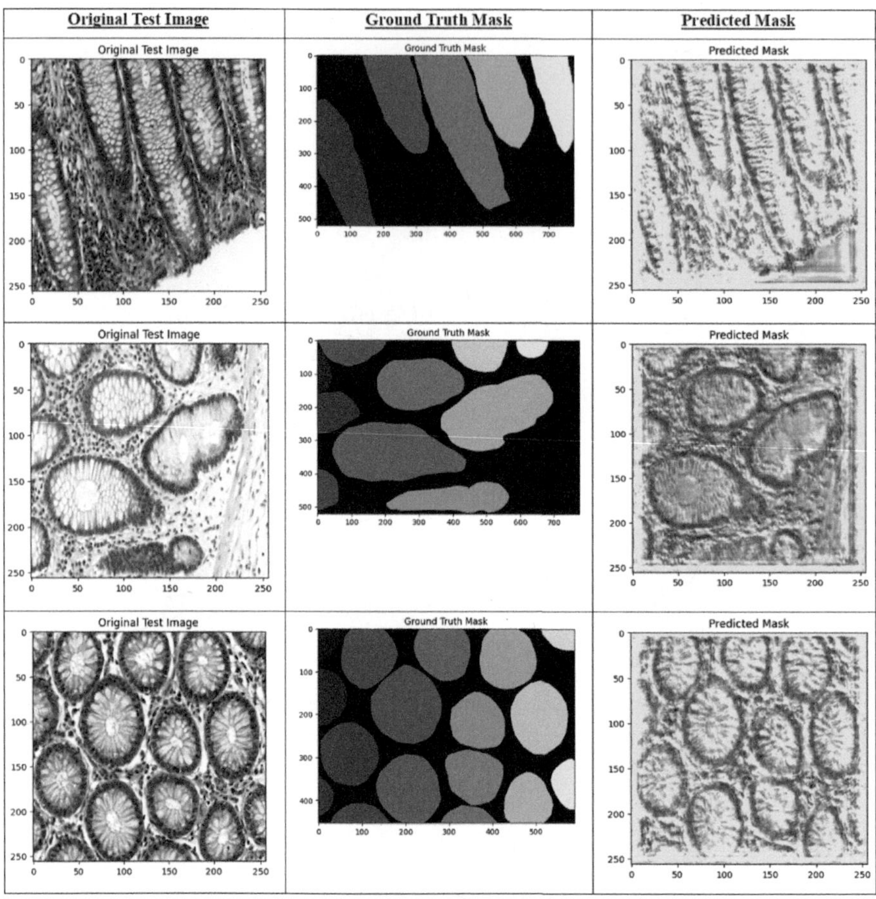

Fig. 5.3   Original test images with their ground truth mask and predicted mask of segmented image

Intersection over Union (IoU), Dice coefficient, Model loss, Dice loss, Recall, Precision, and Accuracy.

The model is trained on a dataset containing patient samples. A range of callbacks including model checkpointing, learning rate reduction, CSV logging, TensorBoard logging, and early stopping are employed to monitor the training process effectively. With the help of these callbacks, management of the training process becomes effective, and they also ensure optimal model performance. In step eight, model evaluation employs custom metrics and post-processing of predicted masks is undertaken in step nine. Finally, in step ten, the images are segmented by the model trained for medical image segmentation, enabling a comprehensive performance assessment by comparing predicted masks with ground truth masks alongside original images. This systematic method ensures that with every stage, there is an advancement in the development of the model, with a specific focus on medical image analysis.

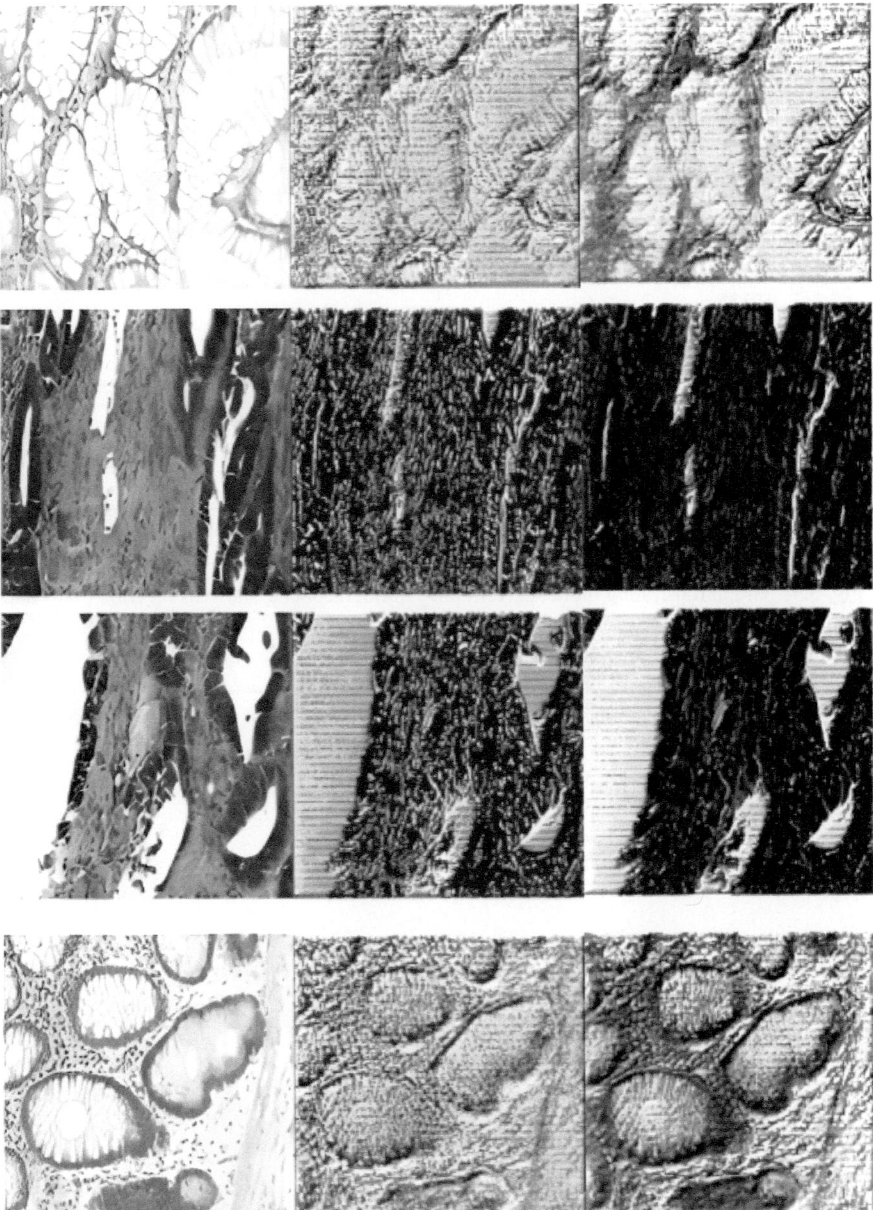

Fig. 5.4 Using a test image to predict a segmentation mask, and then post-processing the mask to visualize the segmented region

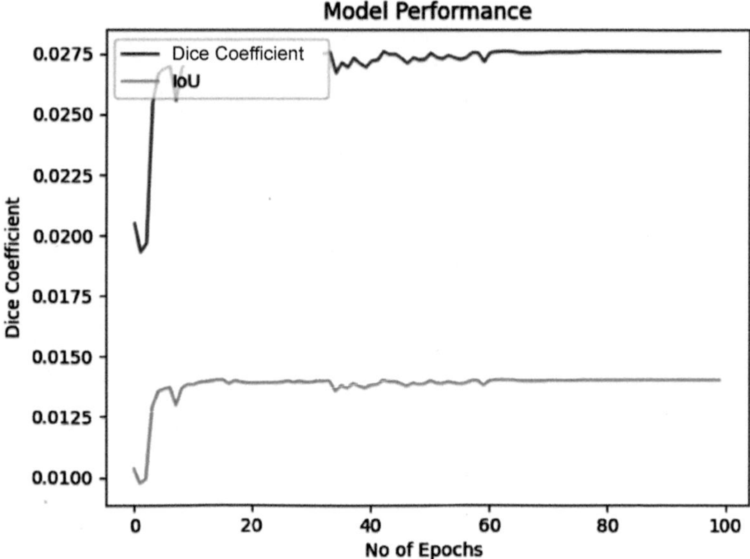

Fig. 5.5   Graph illustrating model performance through epochs, showcasing Dice Coeff and IoU

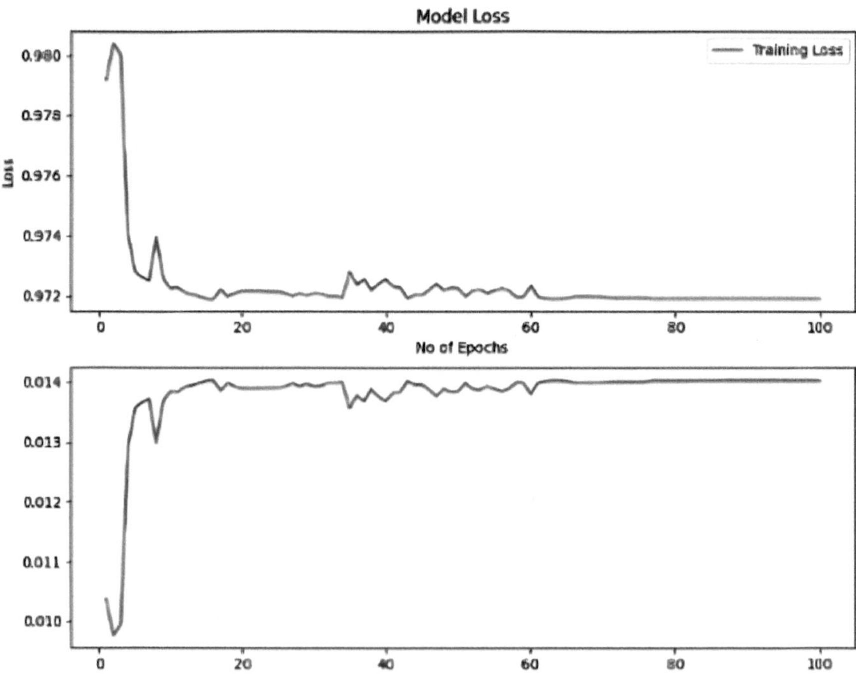

Fig. 5.6   Graph illustrating Model Loss through epochs

Dice Coefficient

$$\text{Dice coefficient} = \frac{2 \times \text{intersection} + \in}{\text{sum (true positive)} + \text{sum (predicted positive)} + \in} \quad ...(1)$$

Intersection over Union (IoU)

$$\text{IoU} = \frac{\text{intersection} + \in}{\text{union} - \text{intersection} + \in} \quad ...(2)$$

Dice Loss

$$\text{Dice Loss} = 1.0 - \text{Dice Coefficient} \quad ...(3)$$

In this instance, the overlapping region—refers to the intersection between the number of true positive and predicted positive elements. Contrary to this, the Union is the total number of elements in both the true positive and predicted positive. For numerical stability, a constant termed epsilon is utilized.

Results

We applied deep learning algorithm-based approaches in this research, specifically utilizing the UNet model architecture and CNNs, for the segmentation of glands in histological images of the colon. By the completion of the entire evaluation using diverse metrics, this method performs remarkably. The segmentation results display absolute accuracy, precision, recall, and F1-score values, indicating the ability of the model to precisely identify glandular structures in histological images with the help of this method. The UNet-based approach effectively captures every complicated detail of the gland boundaries, even in challenging images with overlapping structures.

Conclusion

This research underscores the effectiveness of deep learning methods, particularly the UNet model, in the realm of colon histology image analysis. Achieving accurate gland segmentation holds significant promise for improving diagnostic accuracy and aiding in pathological research related to colon diseases. Our findings emphasize the potential deep learning approaches to revolutionize the analysis of medical images, paving the way for more precise and efficient diagnostic tools. As we continue to advance in this field, integrating deep learning methods into medical imaging processes can significantly enhance our understanding of complex diseases, which will result in better patient results and advancing medical and diagnostic research.

References

Colorectal Cancer Statistics | How Common Is Colorectal Cancer? 2023. American Cancer Society. https://www.cancer.org/cancer/types/colon-rectal-cancer/about/key-statistics.html

Sirinukunwattana, K., Pluim, J.P., Chen, H., Qi, X., Heng, P.A et al., 2017. Gland segmentation in colon histology images: The glas challenge contest. *Medical image analysis*, 35, pp.489–502.

Hamida, A.B., Devanne, M., Weber, J., Truntzer, C., Derangère, V et al., 2021. Deep learning for colon cancer histopathological images analysis. *Computers in Biology and Medicine*, 136, p.104730.

Kainz, P. Pfeiffer M. and Urschler M. 2017. Segmentation and classification of colon glands with deep convolutional neural networks and total variation regularization. PeerJ. 5:e3874. doi: 10.7717/peerj.3874. PMID: 29018612; PMCID: PMC5629961.

Khazaee Fadafen, M. and Rezaee, K., 2023. Ensemble-based multi-tissue classification approach of colorectal cancer histology images using a novel hybrid deep learning framework. *Scientific Reports*, 13(1), p.8823.

Tharwat, M., Sakr, N.A., El-Sappagh, S., Soliman, H., Kwak et al., 2022. Colon Cancer Diagnosis Based on Machine Learning and Deep Learning: Modalities and Analysis Techniques. *Sensors*, 22(23):9250-9250. doi: 10.3390/s22239250.

Rezaei, S., Emami, A., Zarrabi, H., Rafiei, S., Najarian, K. et al., 2019. Gland Segmentation in Histopathology Images Using Deep Networks and Handcrafted Features. arXiv: *Image and Video Processing*.

Nasir, E.S., Parvaiz, A. and Fraz, M.M., 2023. Nuclei and glands instance segmentation in histology images: a narrative review. *Artificial Intelligence Review*, 56:7909-7964. doi: 10.1007/s10462-022-10372-5.

Dabass, M., Vashisth, S. and Vig, R., 2021. Attention-Guided deep atrous-residual U-Net architecture for automated gland segmentation in colon histopathology images. *Informatics in Medicine Unlocked*, 27:100784-. doi: 10.1016/J.IMU.2021.100784

Kosov, A., Khvostikov, A. and Krylov, A., 2020. Adaptive method of glands segmentation on histological images. 2744:1-12. doi: 10.51130/GRAPHICON-2020-2-3-39.

Hamida, A.B., Devanne, M., Weber, J., Truntzer, C., Derangère, V. et al., 2021. Deep learning for colon cancer histopathological images analysis.. *Computers in Biology and Medicine*, 136:104730-. doi: 10.1016/J.COMPBIOMED.2021.104730.

Davri, A., Birbas, E., Kanavos, T., Ntritsos, G., Giannakeas, N et al., 2022. Deep Learning on Histopathological Images for Colorectal Cancer Diagnosis: A Systematic Review. Diagnostics, 12(4):837-837. doi: 10.3390/diagnostics12040837

Hamad, A., Bunyak, F. and Ersoy, I., 2017. Nucleus Classification in Colon Cancer H&E Images using Deep Learning. Microscopy and Microanalysis, 23:1376-1377. doi: 10.1017/S1431927617007541.

Sirinukunwattana, K., Pluim, J.P., Chen, H., Qi, X., Heng, P.A. et al., 2017. Gland Segmentation in Colon Histology Images: The GlaS Challenge Contest. arXiv: *Computer Vision and Pattern Recognition*,

Sirinukunwattana, K., Snead, D.R. and Rajpoot, N.M., 2015. A Stochastic Polygons Model for Glandular Structures in Colon Histology Images. *IEEE Transactions on Medical Imaging*, 34(11):2366-2378. doi: 10.1109/TMI.2015.2433900.

Adaloglou, N. (2021, April 15). An overview of Unet architectures for semantic segmentation and biomedical image segmentation | AI Summer. AI Summer. https://theaisummer.com/unet-architectures/

K, B. (2021, July 6). U-Net architecture for image segmentation. Paperspace Blog. https://blog.paperspace.com/unet-architecture-image-segmentation/

Zhang, J. (2021, December 12). UNET — Line by line Explanation – towards Data science. Medium. https://towardsdatascience.com/unet-line-by-line-explanation-9b191c76baf5

Kirouane, A. (2022, December 8). U-NET (Convolutional Networks for Biomedical Image Segmentation). https://www.linkedin.com/pulse/u-net-convolutional-networks-biomedical-image-ayoub-kirouane

O'Sullivan, C. (2023, March 9). U-Net Explained: Understanding its Image Segmentation Architecture. Medium. https://towardsdatascience.com/u-net-explained-understanding-its-image-segmentation-architecture-56e4842e313a

Maynard-Reid, M. (2023, March 23). U-Net image segmentation in Keras – PyImageSearch. PyImageSearch. https://pyimagesearch.com/2022/02/21/u-net-image-segmentation-in-keras/

G. (2023, June 8). U-Net Architecture Explained. GeeksforGeeks. https://www.geeksforgeeks.org/u-net-architecture-explained/

Colorectal cancer – statistics. (2023, December 8). Cancer.Net. https://www.cancer.net/cancer-types/colorectal-cancer/statistics

Comparative Analysis for Detecting Cancer in Various Organs using Cellular Automata based Segmentation Technique

Rupashri Barik,[1*] *Prakhar Pipersania,*[2] *Samarpan Chandra,*[2]
Samudraneel Banerjee,[2] *Shalini Basak,*[2] *Shashwat Jha*[2]
and *Nazma B. J. Naskar*[3]

The motive of this work is to analyze, examine, review, categorize, and address developments in the human body on cancer detection in several organs using the Cellular Automata based image segmentation technique and machine learning techniques followed by a comparative study. In this work, cancer detection has been done for the brain, breast, cervical region, lips, tongue, chest, and skin. Cancer is a fatal disease that may be inherited from the ancestors and a variety of pathological changes . Early detection of cancer is required and accurate detection is important in order to determine what treatments might be effective in curing it. By identifying cancer at an earlier stage and with more precision, efficient algorithms can save more lives. Here, various medical images of the mentioned organs are being examined and the regions of aberrant cell growth have been identified and the image sets for different organs have been prepared with all the transformed images. Applying different classification techniques on these images, automated

[1]   JIS College of Engineering, WB, India.
[2]   KIIT University, Odisha, India.
[3]   JIS University, WB, India.
*   Corresponding author: barikrupashri@gmail.com

detection of cancer has been performed and the accuracy has been observed. Hence a comparative study has been made between the analysis report obtained for the transformed image set and the analysis report obtained for the original image set for the mentioned cancer.

Introduction

Cancer is a regular cause of demise in the present world. A vast range of diseases arise from aberrant cells dividing quickly and spreading to other tissues and organs. Tumors may be caused by these quickly developing cells. The normal functioning of the body can be disrupted by these. Every day, cancer experts work tirelessly to evaluate new cancer treatments. An automated system for cancer detection may help in this aspect. The physician can detect cancers in various organs more accurately with the help of this automated system much faster. Cancers are named based on their starting area and cell type, even if they spread to other parts of the body. Some specific types of cancers are brain cancer, skin cancer, breast cancer, cervical cancer, liver cancer, oral cancers and lung cancer. Early detection of cancer is very important and an early diagnosis occurs when the cancer is seen in its early stages. This has the potential to improve therapeutic efficacy and reduce mortality. Cancer screenings may help discover cancer symptoms earlier. Some of the most popular cancer screenings may detect:

- Cervical cancer and prostate cancer – Some cancer screenings, such as those for prostate and cervical cancer, may be performed as part of routine checkups.
- Lung cancer – Lung cancer monitoring may be conducted on a regular basis for individuals having specific risk factors.
- Skin cancer – A dermatologist may perform skin cancer screenings for individuals having skin issues or are at risk of skin cancer.
- Breast cancer – Mammograms to check for breast cancer are suggested for women aged 45 and above. However, testing can begin at the age of 40. Testing may be recommended early to the high risk individuals.

While identifying cancer, symptoms can help patients with cancer seek diagnosis and treatment. Some cancers are more difficult to detect early and may not exhibit symptoms until later stages.

AI is now being used more frequently by medical practitioners for detecting cancer. Researchers have discovered that AI can detect and identify colon cancer as well as or better than pathologists using machine learning software by analyzing tissue scans. A team of researchers compared the machine learning technique to the labor of pathologists following the creation of a performance measurement tool. According to the study, most pathologists achieve an accuracy of approximately 0.969 in identifying colon cancer, while the method mentioned here yielded a 0.98 accuracy, indicating more effective results than manual determination.

Existing technologies can also benefit from AI advancements in order to improve patient feedback. Medical practitioners may utilize AI methodologies to quickly and accurately screen chest MRI images in patients with dense breast tissue to exclude those without malignancy, according to a recent study. Although mammography helps reduce breast cancer-related deaths, it is less sensitive in women with exceptionally dense breast tissue. The technique can dramatically reduce radiologists' workload and enhance patient outcomes by merging mammography capabilities with AI.

Background Study

In cancer treatment, predictive models have become indispensable. Predictive models can evaluate an individual's likelihood of acquiring certain malignancies by recognizing risk factors. Patients can then be encouraged to participate in preventive care measures by medical experts. Predictive models assist in decision-making and are very effective in this regard.

Image Segmentation

The importance of time in diagnosing the patient's illness as soon as possible is critical. It can be used to detect a variety of malignant tumors, including brain tumors, breast cancer, and lung cancer. The image segmentation (Kari. 2013) technique performs a crucial function in diagnosing malignancies in several organs. Image segmentation is an important part mostly in the analysis of images, since it allows the splitting of the entire image into distinguished parts based on different objects or regions. The goal of image segmentation is to turn the medical image into a remarkably modified image that can be analyzed effortlessly. Image segmentation is mostly used to recognize objects as well as their edges or limits. The technique of image segmentation may employ the notion of edge detection because it focuses on boundary detection. Thresholding is also significant in image segmentation as it depends on the quality of the input images. Segmentation is conspicuous if the threshold value is higher.

Cellular Automata

Cellular automata are a computational tool which can be used for image processing purposes also due to its uniformity and homogeneity (Gonzalez. 2002). CA rules give better outcomes according to calculation time and explicitness when determining borders along with items of interest present in medical images. The properties of 2D CA are highly suitable for processing images. Using the CA segmentation approach, the area of interest can be divided more effectively. In order to detect the infected area, various transition rules features may be extracted from a variety of image formats.

Figure 6.1 shows the structure of 2-dimensional CA with two different neighborhood models — Von Neumann neighborhood and Moore Neighborhood models. Different operations can be performed on an image using these neighborhood concepts to get a better output image.

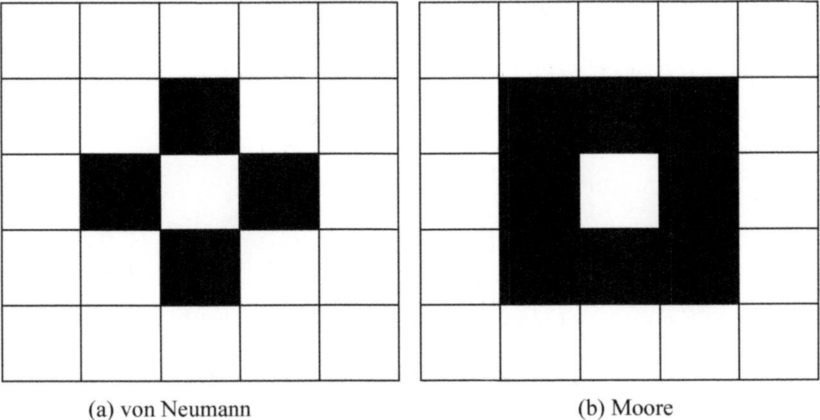

(a) von Neumann　　　　　　　　　　　(b) Moore

Fig. 6.1　2D cellular automata

Cancer Detection

Cancer is a life-threatening disease commonly found in human beings. Growth of abnormal cells in different organs causes cancer. It can be malignant or benign. Early recognition of cancer may reduce the chances of life risk. Initially it can be found as a tumor in different organs. The different types of cancer found in human beings are as follows.

Oral Cancer (Lips & Tongue)

Oral cancer grows on the tongue, under the tongue as well as the base of the tongue and the region of the throat at the back of the mouth. It can also spread to the lips and cheeks. It is also known as mouth cancer which may be caused due to infection or tobacco consumption. It can be cured if it is detected in early stages.

Figure 6.2 are some images showing the pictures of normal mouth and those pictures with a variety of oral cancers.

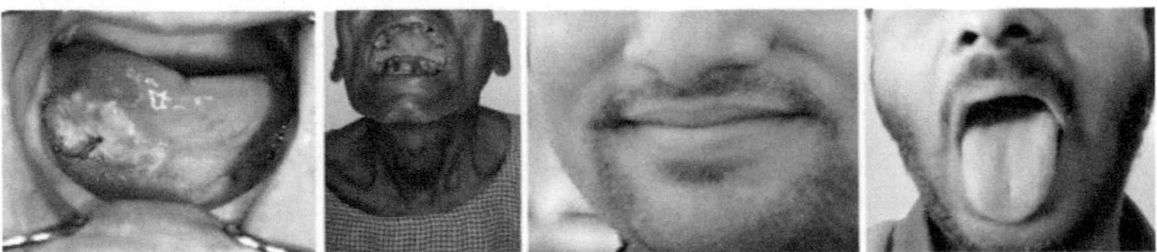

Fig. 6.2　Sample image of normal mouth & oral cancer

Cervical Cancer

Cervical cancer is a growing health concern and a leading cause of loss of life in women. Cervical cancer develops in the cervix's tissue. It is caused by abnormal cell growth that has escalated to other segments of the body. When an automatic detection technique is used to detect precancerous or cancerous cells in a cervical abnormality, no pathologist is required. The detection of cervical cancer cells has played a critical role in clinical practice.

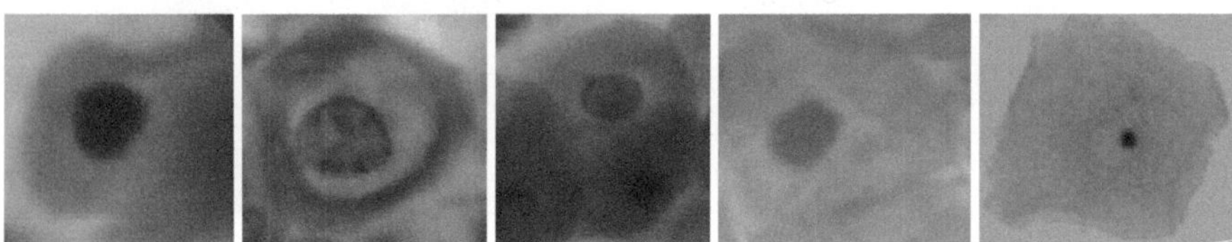

Fig. 6.3 Sample image of cervical cancer

Here Figure 6.3 shows some of the images of cervical cancer in different forms.

Lung Cancer

Lung cancer (He. 2016) is found in the lungs. Cancer from different organs may also spread to the lungs. Cigarette smoking may be the main reason behind it. It is the third most common cancer and it also can be cured if it is detected in the early stage.
Figure 6.4 is a sample of different imaging modalities with lung cancer.

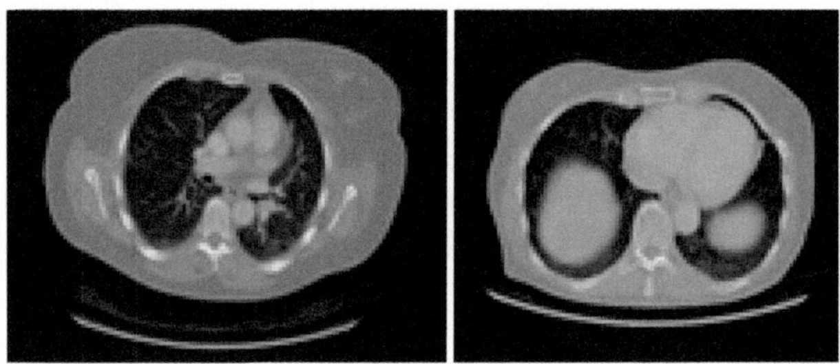

Fig. 6.4 Sample image of normal lungs & lung cancer

Brain Tumor

There are various irregularities in locations and sizes of the brain tumors. It makes a complete understanding of the tumor's nature immensely hard. Analysis of MRI images also necessitates the presence of a qualified neurosurgeon. Often, in developing countries, a lack of skilled doctors and a lack of knowledge about tumors makes generating reports from MRI extremely difficult and time-consuming. A brain tumor is a harmful disease that can affect human beings. Of all primary CNS cancers, 85 to 90 percent are brain tumors. Around 11,700 people are being detected with brain tumors every year. The 5-year success rate for individuals with a central nervous system or malignant brain is around 36% for women and 34%

for men. There exist different categories for brain tumors, including malignant, benign, pituitary, and others. The patients' future ought to be extended by utilizing proper consideration, prior arrangement, and exact determination. The most efficient method for identifying brain tumors is MRI. The scans provide a massive quantity of image data. The pathologist looks over the medical imaging. As brain tumors and their characteristics are so complicated, a manual assessment can be prone to errors. Appropriate care, preparation, and precise diagnosis should be used to extend patients' lives. The best method for finding brain cancers is MRI. A huge amount of picture information is produced from the scan images. The radiologist examines these images. A manual investigation can be prone to mistakes because of the complexity of brain tumors and characteristics.

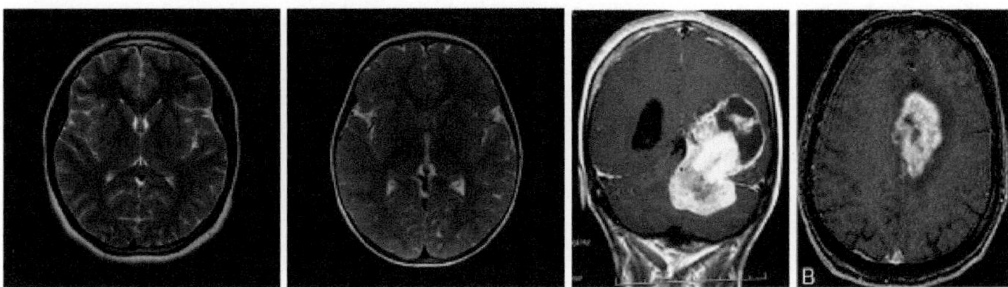

Fig. 6.5   Sample image of normal brain & brain tumor

Figure 6.5 shows some sample images of brain tumors. The first two images are the CT-scan images of the normal brain and the latter two are the imaging modalities with brain tumor.

Predictive Models Assist Decision Making

More precisely, deep learning can distinguish between mammograms taken from women who will develop breast cancer later on and those taken from women who will not. Mammograms can not only help diagnose cancer, but they can also predict the risk of breast cancer by analyzing breast density. While dense breasts on mammography are typically associated with a higher risk of cancer, other unknown characteristics concealed in the mammogram could also contribute to the risk. Because of the high costs of treatment and the uncertainty of a patient's cure, making medical decisions about a cancer diagnosis can be particularly difficult. By aggregating data insights, a less expensive and speedier means of predicting whether a person would be impacted by cancer, as well as aiding in early diagnosis and treatment, can be achieved. Cancer screening can also help patients have a better post-cancer physical condition and decrease treatment expenditures.

With large amounts of medical data being collected, there is a pressing need to make efficient use of this data in order to enhance the health-care sector worldwide. Only recent research may be utilized to examine the deep learning and machine learning models currently in use for medical data. In the medical field, deep learning methodologies are gaining traction over machine learning methods, signaling a shift in how artificial intelligence is used. In this section different predictive models are described.

CNN 2D Model and ANN-Combined Model

CNN's extraordinary learning ability mostly stems from its usage of a variety of component extraction services, which allow it to subsequently extract representations from the data. The analysis of CNNs has accelerated due to increased information accessibility and equipment innovation (Kumar. 2019), and recently, novel deep CNN designs have been reported. Several exciting strategies for obtaining more advanced CNNs have been studied, such as the application of different enactment and misfortune capacities, boundary streamlining, regularization, and compositional advancements.

In Figure 6.6 the CNN and ANN models have been illustrated as they have been used in the proposed work. It represents a combined model based on the concept of CNN and ANN.

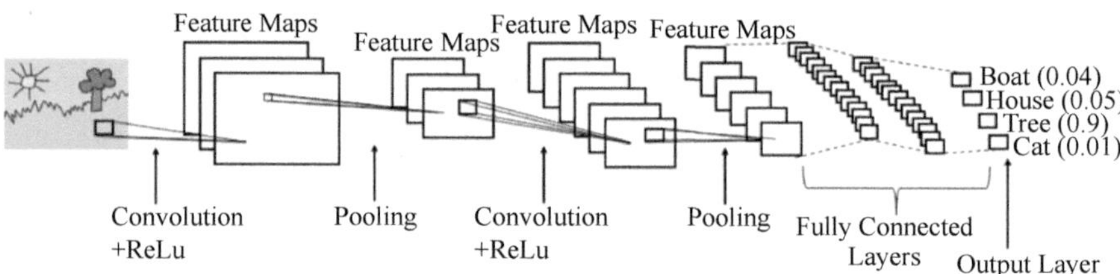

Fig. 6.6　CNN & ANN – combined model

(a) CNN: Convolution Neural Networks typically require more input data to achieve their high accuracy rates effectively (Barik. 2021). CNN's primary benefit is that it can identify key traits automatically without human oversight. For this reason, CNN would be the perfect answer to issues with picture classification and computer vision. Feature maps generated after using convolutional layers take a part of the image, which is then split into rectangles and transferred to nonlinear processing. The initial layer in the process of removing attributes from an input image is called convolution. With the use of learning visual traits with little squares of information, convolution protects the connection between pixels. A kernel or filter and an image matrix are the two inputs to this mathematical process. Next, attribute selection, uses the filters with strides, and padding as needed. ReLU activation is to be applied to the matrix after convoluting the picture. While the image size is very large, the layer pooling portion would reduce the number of layers. Spatial Pooling (known as sub-pooling or down sampling) reduces the size of each map, while preserving major details. Spatial pooling is of various types:

- Sum Pooling
- Average Pooling
- Max Pooling

Max pooling uses the maximum component of the corrected feature map. Selecting the highest element may cause the average to pool. Total pooling involves the amount of all components in an element map.

(b) ANN: An artificial neural network (ANN) is the perfect solution for data-related problems. The forward-facing algorithm can easily handle image, text, and table data. An ANN transmits information in one direction traversing through various input nodes until it reaches the output node. Hidden layers within the network may exist, facilitating the network's operations with clarity. In the proposed model, the inputs consist of images that have been transformed and scaled to dimensions of 64×64 for all models, and specifically for the model related to cervical [cancer]. Then the feature map is built followed by the addition of convolution and max pooling layers with specific filter values. Next, layers related to the output dim (size of dense embedding) of 128 were created with rectilinear activation characteristics. Additionally, express go entropy has been utilized to calculate the loss. Therefore, the error is computed in the output layer using softmax activation characteristics, and the adam optimizer is repeatedly applied through the network to adjust its parameters and improve performance. Here the proposed model is a mix of CNN & ANN. They have their own advantages & disadvantages so we attempted to create a model that would integrate the advantages of both while minimizing the drawbacks.

VGG Model

VGG16 is one of the famous convolution neural network (CNN) architectures in the deep learning field. The most distinct feature of VGG16 is its design with a large number of hyper-parameters. It utilizes convolutional layers with 3×3 filters, a stride of 1, and typically employs the same padding.Additionally, it includes maxpooling layers with 2×2 filters and a stride of 2. Throughout the architecture, this association of max pool and convolution layers is consistent. Eventually, it has FC (completely related layers) and a softmax layer for getting output. The sixteen in VGG16 implies having sixteen layers with weights. The network is quite large, containing approximately 138 million parameters. Training it required several weeks and utilized NVIDIA Titan Black GPUs.

Here, Figure 6.7 illustrates the used VGG model. In this work, VGG accepts a 256×256 RGB picture. To maintain consistency with the input image size required for the ImageNet competition, the creators cropped out the centeral 256×256 patch in each image. The convolutional layers of VCG have a relatively small receptive field (3×3, which is the minimum size required to capture information both vertically and horizontally). There are additional 1×1 convolution filters applied to the input image, which perform a linear transformation of the input before passing through a ReLU unit. A convolution stride is set at a pixel to keep up with the spatial goal next to convolution. The three fully connected layers of VGG consist of 1000 channels, one for individual classes, in the first two layers, each with 4096 channels. ReLU is utilized by all of VGG's hidden layers (A huge upgrade from

AlexNet that reduces training time). It doesn't utilize Local Response Normalisation (LRN) in general as it expands memory consumption and time for training with no discernible gain in accuracy.

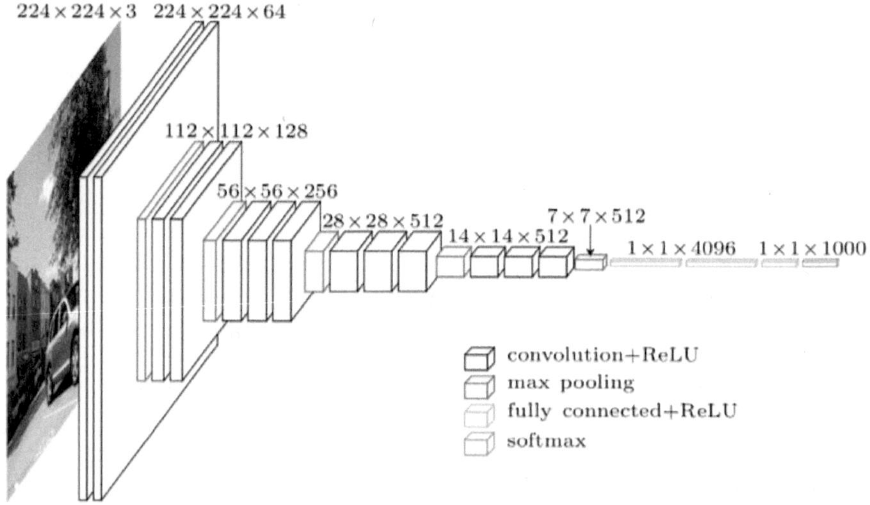

Fig. 6.7   VGG architecture

ResNet-50 Model

ResNet-50 is a deep convolutional neural network with 50 layers, utilized in various medical imaging tasks such as cervical cancer detection (SipakMed, 2021), chest CT scan image analysis (2020), brain tumor detection (2022), oral cancer detection from images of lips and tongue, 2020). A pre-educated model of the community educated on over one million snapshots can be loaded from the ImageNet database. The pretrained community can categorize snap shots into one thousand special item categories, inclusive of keyboards, mice, pencils, and quite a few animals. As a consequence, the community has learnt special attributes and depictions for a numerous set of pictures. The network features a 256 × 256 picture input size.

Inception Model

Inception internet accomplished a milestone in CNN classifiers while preceding fashions had been simply going deeper to enhance the overall performance and accuracy however compromising the computational cost. The Inception network, on the other hand, is closely engineered. It makes use of a number of hints to push overall performance, each in phrases of velocity and accuracy. Although preceding networks along with VGG accomplished top notch accuracy at the ImageNet dataset, deploying those sorts of fashions is notably computationally costly due to the deep architecture. Huge deep networks also are vulnerable to overfitting. It seems difficult to pass gradient updates through the complete network. As a result, Inception was picked as one of the models to test on the cancer datasets and make the comparison with the proposed algorithm and model.

R. Barik et al., (Barik. 2021a) proposed a mechanism for detecting various cancers in different organs. This work utilizes the cellular automata-based segmentation technique for detecting cancer in various organs. Applying the Moore neighborhood concept, image segmentation has been performed to distinguish the region of abnormal mass growth from its background image. Here various imaging modalities like brain CT-Scan, breast mammography and chest X-ray have been considered for detecting tumors in the brain, breast and lungs, respectively. In addition to this approach, the author has proposed a predictive model (Simonyan. 2014) for determining covid infection in human lungs. This predictive model is a combination of CNN and ANN using which automatic detection of COVID-19 infection occurs. Here, the proposed CA-based segmentation method is applied initially to perform image segmentation, separating the infected area from the background of chest X-rays. Subsequently, a new set of images is prepared and trained using the proposed training model to automatically detect COVID-19 infections.

Extending the idea of the CA-based image segmentation technique, here a comparative analysis has been made for the performance measurement of detecting different cancers in various organs. The proposed CA-based total image segmentation approach has been implemented to create a distinctive image set of numerous organs like brain, lung, spine, lips and tongue to segment the different infected areas from their background for detecting brain tumor, lung cancer, cervical cancer and oral cancer respectively. With the obtained transformed images, a new image set of various cancers have been prepared and different predictive models have been applied to these newly obtained images set for measuring performance. These results have been compared with the performance measured for the various cancer image sets without applying the CA-based image segmentation technique.

Methodology

In this section the working procedure has been discussed briefly. Here two steps have been followed. In the first step, image segmentation has been performed using the cellular automata-based technique followed by performance measurement done subsequent to the application of various image classifications algorithms.

Illustration of CA-based Image Segmentation Algorithm
Step 1: Input image
Step 2: Enhancing quality of the image using bilateral filter
Step 3: Padding the enhanced image with 0
Step 4: Image segmentation using Moore Neighborhood operation of cellular automata
Step 5: Set a threshold value based on input image

Step 6: Obtain negative image
Step 7: Get the binary image
Step 8: Obtain transformed image

Cancer images of various organs have been taken as the input here. After enhancing the quality of the input X-ray or CT image, the Moore neighborhood concept of Cellular Automata has been applied as a transition rule for separating the growth of mass from its background found in different organs. All eight of the surrounding cells are subtracted from the single central cell that has been examined. If the variations are much less than the selected threshold, then the value of the reference cell gets changed to 0, otherwise it remains the same. The threshold value has been chosen based on the input image. Then the obtained image has been inverted and finally image binarization has been performed to obtain the segmented image.

In the next stage, predictive models have been used to make the decision of accuracy on the basis of different performance measures. For this, different image sets of various cancers have been considered from different online sources. Following are the steps for measuring the accuracy of cancer detection in various organs.

Data Retrieval/Pre-processing

The dataset is imported from Kaggle and copied to the newly processed folder. Iterate over the images in the folder, reading them, resizing them to 256×256, and applying a 2×2 average blur filter. Write a new name for the image based on its class and delete the old one. We'll delete the duplicate images from the dataset because there are a lot of them. It is being iterated through all of the other images in the folder to remove the duplicate. Then, in grayscale mode, it will discover the root mean square value for both the image and if it is less than 3, which is an empirically determined value the duplicate image will be removed from the folder. The dataset is copied to the newly processed folder. And go to all the images in the folder, reading them, resizing the image to 256×256, padding the image by 2px on each side, applying a 2×2 average blur filter, and renaming the image based on its class, and deleting the previous image. Hence, the discussed image segmentation technique has been applied.

Data Expansion

The Keras ImageDataGenerator class has the advantage of being designed for real-time data augmentation i.e., while the model is in training, it is creating augmented images on the go. At each epoch, the ImageDataGenerator class ensures that the model gets new picture variants. It only delivers the edited images and does not include them in the actual image corpus. For such cases, the model would be repeatedly revealed to the original images, plainly outstripping the model here.

Model training with various models

To compare the processed output with sample output, the training model uses the algorithm to process input data. Over varied threshold ranges, CNN, VGG, Inception, and Resnet are used. Optimizer, Max Epochs, Learning Rate, Dropout Rate, Batch Size, and other parameters are necessary for training the CNN Model. Learning rate, Loss Function, Optimizer, and Metrics are needed parameters for training the VGG Model. The optimization approach and the learning rate schedule are needed parameters for training the Inception. Learning rate, number of epochs, and batch size are needed parameters for training the Resnet Model.

Evaluation of the model

This involves calculating evaluation metrics for characteristics like accuracy, validation accuracy, validation loss, and presenting graphs for the analysis for multiple threshold values such as 100, 150, 200, and 250. After transformation, multiple images are trained with the proposed methodology in order to develop an automated system for recognizing infection automatically. Transformed images were scaled to 256×256 pixels and multiplied with multiple feature detectors with a stride of 1 and with rectilinear activation function to extract the finest feature from the transformed image, yielding two alternative feature maps. Then, to minimize the size of the image matrix, multiply the 3×3 feature detector with a big matrix of 256×256 input pictures. Following that, max pooling was performed, and a 2×2 pixel box was considered and set in the top left corner. Now it is necessary to determine the highest value in that box, which will be decreased. Then the box is shifted to the right side with a two-step stride. In this case, maximum pooling was used to minimize the size of the 32 individual feature maps, yielding 32 pooled feature maps. Three additional convolution layers are appended to the train and test set to improve accuracy. The first one uses a three-by-three matrix of 32 feature detectors. The second uses a 3×3 matrix with 64 feature detectors, while the third uses a 3×3 matrix with 128 feature detectors. Max pooling was applied to individual convolution layers going forward. Now flatten the individual pooled feature map into a column. Simply add the numbers from the pooled feature map to a single long column to create a single large vector of inputs for an ANN. The converted image set is resized before being used as the convolution layer's input. Then two completely connected layers with output dim (density of dense embedding) of 128 were created, and the loss was calculated using categorical cross entropy with a rectilinear activation function. As a result, error is computed at the output layer using the softmax activation function followed by back propagation through the network using the Adam optimizer to change the network and improve performance. The ANN concept has been used in this case. Three hidden layers were investigated in this section, and eventually, the output image was obtained from the completely linked layer, which detects infections.

Required Image Set

For the experimental setup, image sets of various cancers are required and following are the details of the image sets which have been considered for further discussion.

Oral Cancer (Lips & Tongue)

For oral cancer, the image classification dataset has been collected from various hospitals in Ahmedabad and classified with the assistance of ENT doctors. It includes images of the tongue and lips that have been classified as cancerous or non-cancerous. 87 images of cancer and 44 non-Cancer images have been considered here.

Cervical Cancer

The SipakMed database contains 4049 images of isolated cells that were manually cropped from 966 cluster cell images of Pap smear slides. The images were captured using an optical microscope and a CCD camera. Abnormal, normal and benign cells are divided into five categories in the cell images as follows:

- Dyskeratotic (813 Isolated cells) - (223 Cluster Cell)
- Koilocytotic (825 Isolated cells) - (238 Cluster Cell)
- Metaplastic (793 Isolated cells) - (271 Cluster Cell)
- Parabasal (787 Isolated cells) - (108 Cluster Cell)
- Superficial-Intermediate (831 Isolated cells) - (126 Cluster Cell)

Chest CT-Scan

Using an AI model, the dataset can be used to classify and identify whether a patient has cancer or not. The image set was taken from Kaggle. These datasets include three types of chest cancer: squamous cell carcinoma, adenocarcinoma, large cell carcinoma, and normal cell. The image set has been split as follows for the training purpose.

- Training Set: 70%
- Testing Set: 20%
- Validation Set: 10%
- Squamous cell carcinoma: Squamous cell lung cancer develops amongst major airway branches or centrally in the lung, where the larger bronchi join the trachea to the lung. Around 30% of non-small cell lung cancers are squamous cell lung cancers that are frequently linked to smoking. The final folder contains the standard CT-Scan images.
- Adenocarcinoma: The most frequent form of lung cancer, lung adenocarcinoma, represents 40% of cases of non-small cell lung cancer and 30% of all cases. Numerous cancers, such as colorectal, prostate, and breast cancers, can have adenocarcinomas. It is found in the glands that secrete mucus and support

breathing in the outer part of the lung. Symptoms include weakness, weight loss, hoarseness, and coughing.

- Large cell carcinoma: Any place in the lung may develop large-cell identical carcinoma lung cancer that spreads swiftly and grows. Ten to fifteen percent of cases of NSCLC are usually of this type of lung cancer. Large-cell carcinoma that is not differentiated grows and spreads swiftly.
- Normal cells: Normal cells represent no growth of abnormal cells which implies no cancerous cells are present in the lungs.

Brain Tumor

The brain tumor image set has been taken from Kaggle with 155 brain tumor images and 98 no-brain tumor images. Following are some sample images of brain tumor and the corresponding transformed images or segmented images of brain tumor with different threshold values.

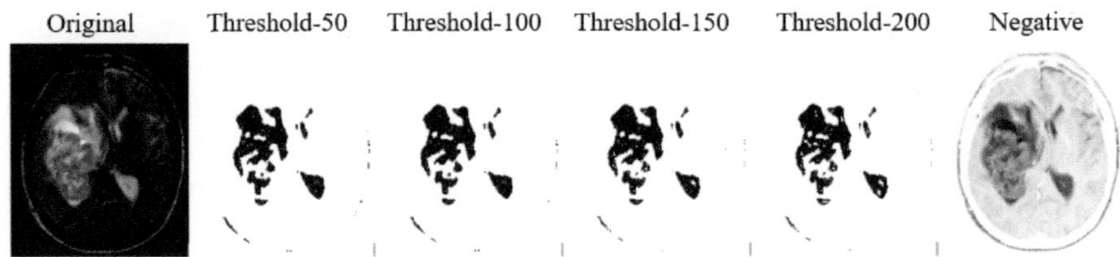

Fig. 6.8   Brain tumor segmentation with different threshold values

Figure 6.8 emphasizes different output images of brain tumors with different threshold values like 50, 100, 150 and 200 respectively. The last image is the negative image for the original image of the brain tumor shown here.

Splitting the Dataset

Splitting of the used image set is much required here. The whole image set has been split into the Train Set, Validation Set & Test Set in the ratio of 70:15:15 respectively. Accordingly, they have been copied to their respective new folders.

Results & Discussions

In this section, a comparative analysis is made for cancer detection in different organs applying the proposed segmentation technique simultaneously with the original image set. Here, the performance measures have been done considering the accuracy and data loss. In Table 6.1, 6.2(a), 6.2(b), 6.2(c), 6.2(d), 6.3(a), 6.3(b), 6.4, 6.5(a) and 6.5(b),that follow, the symbols A and L indicate the model accuracy and the loss respectively.

Table 6.1   Accuracy/loss metrics table with image segmentation

Epochs: 32	Data Split	Threshold	CNN		VGG		Inception		Resnet	
Dataset			A	L	A	L	A	L	A	L
Brain MRI	75:15:15	150	95.99	0.21	83.99	0.34	95.99	1.11	87.99	0.55
Chest CT-Scan	70:10:20	200	25.00	0.56	86.03	0.55	80.95	0.29	83.81	0.19
Oral Lip & Tongue Cancer	70:15:15	150	58.82	0.61	82.35	0.43	76.47	12.63	70.58	0.47
Cervical Cancer	70:15:15	150	90.311	0.260	80.29	0.45	75.04	0.59	53.36	1.18

Table 6.1 illustrates the comparison of the performance measures applying different predictive models to the new transformed image set of various cancers obtained for different threshold values. In the later part, a brief discussion has been made on the comparison of performance measures among cancers in various organs using the predictive models followed by the application of the proposed segmentation technique and without applying any segmentation technique. The following tables illustrate the performance measures for separate image sets of brain tumor, lung cancer, oral cancer and cervical cancer after applying various prediction models.

For Brain Image Dataset

Table 6.2(a) shows the performance measures for the brain tumor image set after applying various existing predictive models with the proposed model. All these models are used to create a newly created image set of output images, generated after using the segmentation technique to the brain tumor image set with different threshold values. The data split ratio has been taken as 75:15:10.

Table 6.2(a)   Accuracy/Loss Metrics Table with different Thresholds and with Segmentation Technique

With Segmentation	Threshold	Epochs	CNN+ANN (Proposed)		VGG		Inception		Resnet	
Data Split			A	L	A	L	A	L	A	L
75:15:10	100	32	61.538	0.618	84.615	0.635	84.615	0.35	57.692	0.968
75:15:10	150	32	61.538	0.618	80.769	0.325	80.769	0.33	61.538	0.621
75:15:10	200	32	61.538	0.618	84.615	0.413	76.923	1.594	50	0.601
75:15:10	250	32	61.538	0.618	84.615	0.425	88.461	0.563	73.076	0.986

Table 6.2(b) shows the performance measures for same brain tumor image set after applying different existing predictive models and the proposed model without prior segmentation and here the data split ratio is 75:15:10. It can be observed that the results get better while the transformed images are used.

Table 6.2(b)   Accuracy/loss metrics table with different thresholds without segmentation technique

Without Segmentation		CNN+ANN (Proposed)		VGG		Inception		Resnet	
Data Split	Epochs	A	L	A	L	A	L	A	L
75:15:10	32	61.538	0.655	76.923	0.517	65.384	6.382	61.538	0.895
75:15:10	32	61.538	0.61	88.461	0.275	80.769	0.214	80.769	0.901

Table 6.2(c)   Accuracy/loss metrics table without segmentation technique

Without Segmentation	Epochs	CNN+ANN (Proposed)		VGG		Inception		Resnet	
Data Split		A	L	A	L	A	L	A	L
70:15:15	32	72.00	0.35	83.99	0.34	95.99	1.108	87.99	0.55

Table 6.2(d)   Accuracy/loss metrics table with segmentation technique

With Segmentation	Epochs	Threshold	CNN+ANN (Proposed)	
Data Split			A (Accuracy)	L (Loss)
70:15:15	32	150	95.99	0.21

In Tables 6.2(c) and 6.2(d), additionally, it has been shown that for the data split ratio 70:15:15, the proposed model produced better results considering the new image set of transformed images, obtained after applying segmentation technique to the same brain tumor image set. While the models are applied to the real image set, it results in lower accuracy than the earlier one.

For Oral Cancer (Lips & Tongue)

Table 6.3(a) illustrates the performance measures for the oral cancer image set after applying different existing predictive models with the proposed model. All these models are used to create a new image set of output images, obtained after using the segmentation technique to the oral cancer image set with different threshold values.

Table 6.3(a)   Accuracy/loss metrics table with different thresholds and with segmentation technique

With Segmentation	Threshold	Epochs	CNN		VGG		Inception		Resnet	
Data Split			A	L	A	L	A	L	A	L
70:15:15	100	32	58.82	0.512	76.47	0.29	70.59	1.3847	64.7	0.84
70:15:15	150	32	58.82	0.615	82.35	0.433	76.47	12.633	70.588	0.47
70:15:15	200	32	47.06	0.375	76.47	0.413	76.47	16.23	64.7	0.953
70:15:15	250	32	58.82	0.658	76.47	0.425	64.7	2.38	70.58	0.83

Table 6.3(b) shows the performance measures for the same oral cancer image set after applying different predictive models and the proposed model without prior segmentation and here the data split ratio is 70:15:10.

Table 6.3(b)   Accuracy/loss metrics table without segmentation technique

Without Segmentation		CNN		VGG		Inception		Resnet	
Data Split	Epochs	A	L	A	L	A	L	A	L
70:15:15	32	47.05	0.622	76.47	0.207	82.35	0.775	70.58	0.497
70:15:15(CNN)	32	70.588	0.58	76.47	0.207	82.35	0.775	70.58	0.497

For Lung Cancer Image set

Table 6.4. illustrates the performance measures for the lung cancer image set considering different predictive models with the proposed model. All the models have been applied to the image set after performing segmentation.

Table 6.4   Accuracy/loss metrics table with different thresholds with segmentation technique

With Segmentation	Threshold	Epochs	CNN+ANN (Proposed)		VGG		Inception		Resnet	
Data Split			A	L	A	L	A	L	A	L
70:10:20	100	32	25	0.562	81.269	0.464	73.333	0.312	79.682	0.578
70:10:20	150	32	25	0.562	78.1	0.465	82.4	0.25	85.4	0.25
70:10:20	200	32	25	0.562	86.031	0.552	80.95	0.292	83.81	0.192
70:10:20	250	32	25	0.562	69.206	0.573	80.634	0.295	78.095	0.178

For Cervical Cancer

Following the same approaches, the performance measures comparison has been shown in Table 6.5(a) for the cervical cancer image set. Different existing predictive models have been used to the newly created image set of transformed images, generated by the segmentation technique with different threshold values.

Table 6.5(a)   Accuracy/loss metrics table with different thresholds with segmentation technique

With Segmentation	Threshold	Epochs	CNN		VGG		Inception		Resnet	
Data Split			A	L	A	L	A	L	A	L
70:15:15	100	32	89.133	0.376	79.01	0.53	76.043	0.418	53.038	1.157
70:15:15	150	32	90.311	0.260	80.29	0.45	75.04	0.59	53.36	1.18
70:15:15	200	32	89.461	0.301	80.101	0.452	75.00	0.508	52.382	1.221
70:15:15	250	32	90.045	0.265	79.55	0.39	71.609	0.508	51.831	1.191

Table 6.5(b) represents the performance measures for the cervical image set after applying different models without prior segmentation with a data split ratio of 75:15:15.

Table 6.5(b)   Accuracy/loss metrics table without segmentation technique

Without Segmentation	Epochs	CNN		VGG		Inception		Resnet	
Data Split		A	L	A	L	A	L	A	L
70:15:15	32	90.147	0.211	86.04	0.421	78.325	0.54	62.068	1.14

Visual Analysis

The following graphs represent the accuracy comparison for all predictive models applied for the individual cancer image sets.

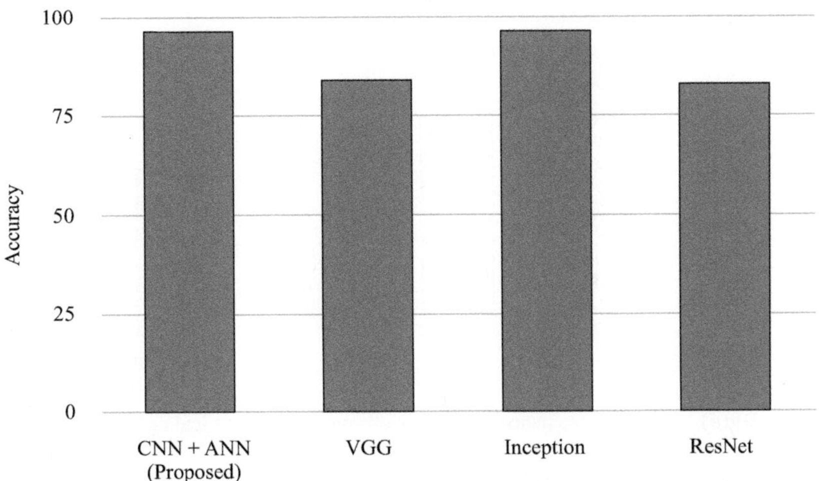

Fig. 6.9(a)   Performance measures for various models for brain tumor image set

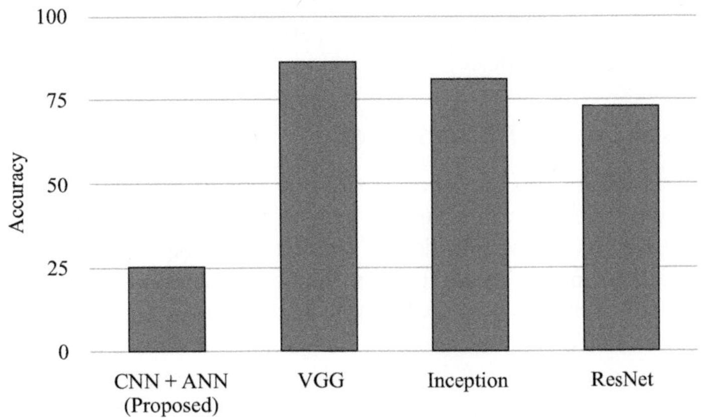

Fig. 6.9(b)   Performance measures for various models for lung cancer image set

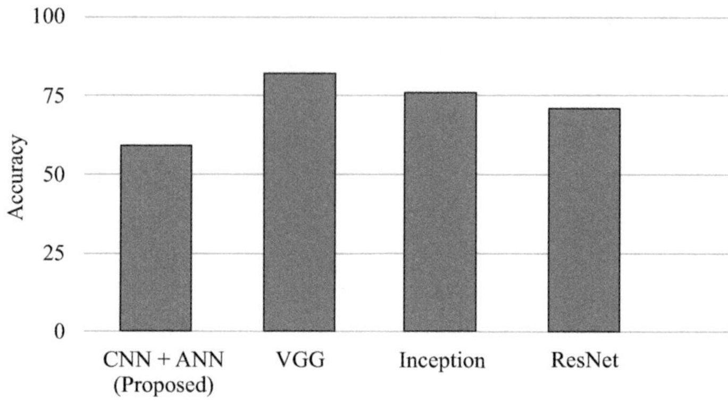

Fig. 6.9(c)   Performance measures for various models for oral cancer image set

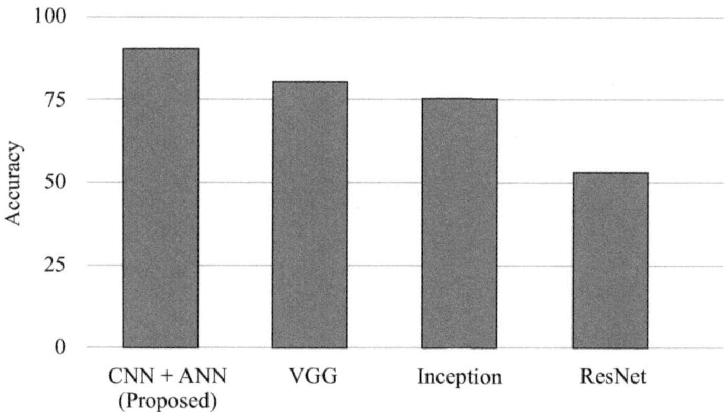

Fig. 6.9(d)   Performance measures for various models for cervical cancer image set

Figures 6.9(a), 6.9(b), 6.9(c) and 6.9(d) are the graphical representations of performance measures for the brain tumor image set, lung cancer image set, oral cancer image set and cervical cancer image set respectively. For all these image sets, the obtained accuracy has been compared for proposed model and VGG, Inception and ResNet mode.

Concerns of Chest CT Scan Dataset

It is essential to discuss the concerns of the image datasets as this model's performance was very low in comparison to the others Deep Learning Models. So here two sets of images are considered. The first set visibly contains the images of the tumor sample and the second one has the normal samples.

Apparently looking at Figure 6.10, at first, it looks as if both the original images are tumorous. Therefore, both the images are very similar in nature resulting in ambiguous predictions of the same. Although after applying binary inversion

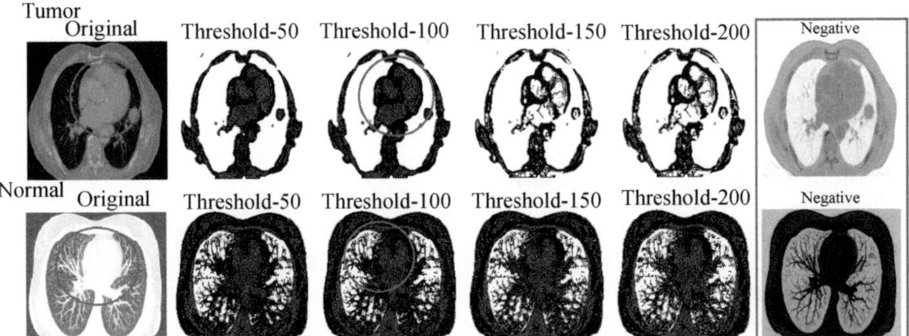

Fig. 6.10   Negative image of brain tumor and normal brain with different threshold values

without the threshold value, we get the negative images. Here, we can easily differentiate between the tumor samples and the cancer unaffected image sample. Another reason for the model to perform poorly may be the application of the Moore neighborhood algorithm which is the proposed technique for processing, applied with threshold values. So, in the tumor samples across different threshold values, we can identify the tumor easily but in the normal samples the effect is seen to be completely opposite as the nerves and parts of the lungs are colored in black indicating them as tumors.

In Figure 6.11, the two images of lungs seem to be completely different but looking at the structure of the lungs it can be observed that only the colors have been inverted showing that there are multiple duplicate images in the dataset. This was one of the prime reasons for getting low accuracy. Finally, the reason may be the distortion and the noise present in the duplicate images which subsequently confuses the proposed techniques as it uses the method of contouring, i.e., highlighting the tumor cells.

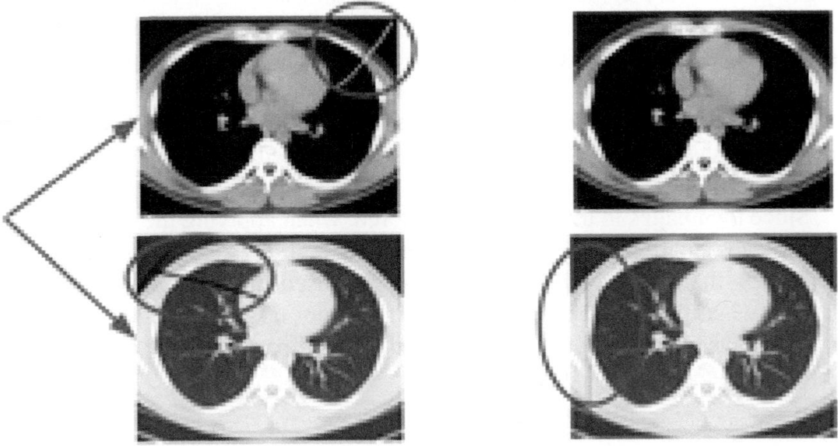

Fig. 6.11   CT–Scan image of lungs

Finally, in the performance analysis, the reasons mentioned amalgamate to the poor accuracy of the proposed model. In contrast, when we don't apply the Moore neighborhood algorithm, the accuracy of the proposed model increases to some extent.

Concerns of Brain MRI Dataset

The tumor can be seen with the naked eye in the first series of images. So when we apply the algorithm, it outlines the tumor in black, assisting the model in identifying the tumorous sample.

In Figure 6.12 the MRI image of brain has been taken and has been transformed to a negative image with threshold values 50, 100, 150 and 200.

In the second set because the light intensities in the image are quite dispersed in the set below, the color of the tumor turns white. This is the inverse color impact of the suggested procedure. So, the tumor appears black in the first image but white in the second. This might confuse the model, lowering its performance. This was one of the reasons we thought about improving the images. Images with similar pixel intensities have been chosen in this refining procedure. Some of the images with incorrect categories were also eliminated. Greater accuracy is obtained in the revised dataset than in the original one despite the fact that the split ratio of the testing dataset has been raised. Another finding was that using segmentation resulted in higher accuracy, whilst not using segmentation resulted in lower accuracy, which serves as proof of the concept for our suggested technique.

Concerns of Oral Cancer Dataset

It is observed that images of oral cancer have many features when compared to those of Brain MRI and Cervical cancer in which the tumor cells are very concentrated. Moore neighborhood algorithm uses contouring which bounds the features of the images. As there are so many features, it detects unnecessary objects which can be seen highlighted in the image such as glasses. As a result the images are wrongly classified. For colored images also the entire approach has been applied. Figure 6.13 shows the color image of a normal mouth and the image of disputed lips. Both the colored images of lip have been converted to negative images with different threshold values 100, 150, 200, 250 and the transformed images have been shown in the Figure 6.13.

Since the images in the dataset are colored, when applying the algorithm, the color spreads and because of that the tumor is not highlighted, and it disseminates. The causes that were cited add up to the proposed model's low accuracy. In contrast, when the segmentation algorithm was not used and trained the model for numerous iterations, it achieved an accuracy comparable to the other Transfer Learning Models.

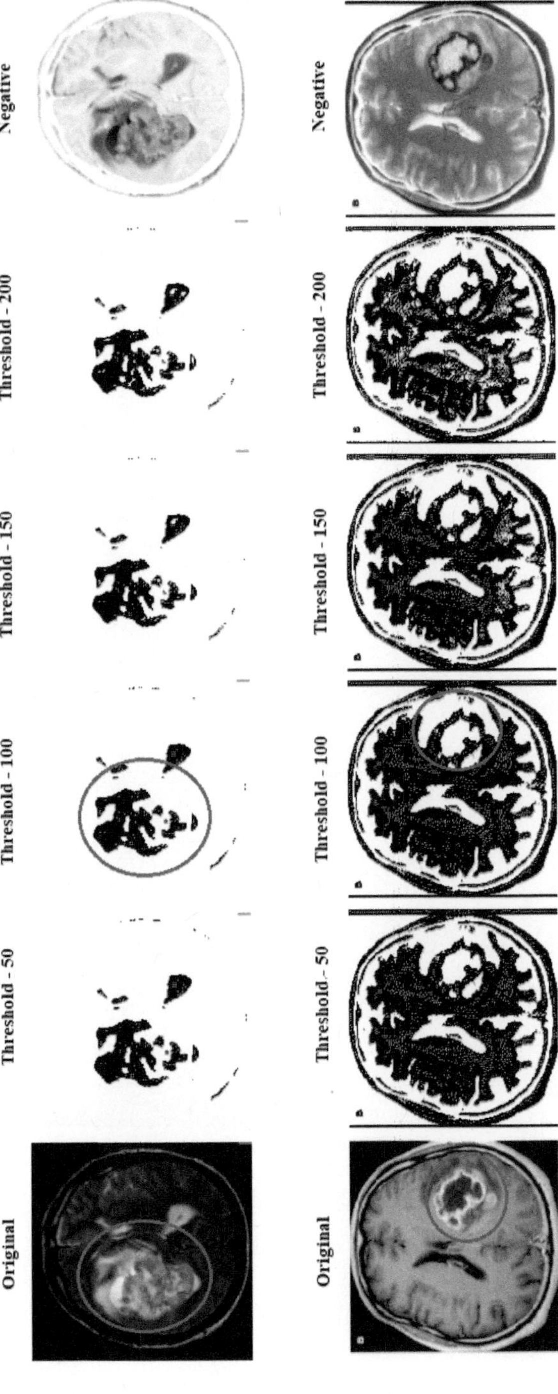

Fig. 6.12   Negative image of brain MRI image with different threshold values

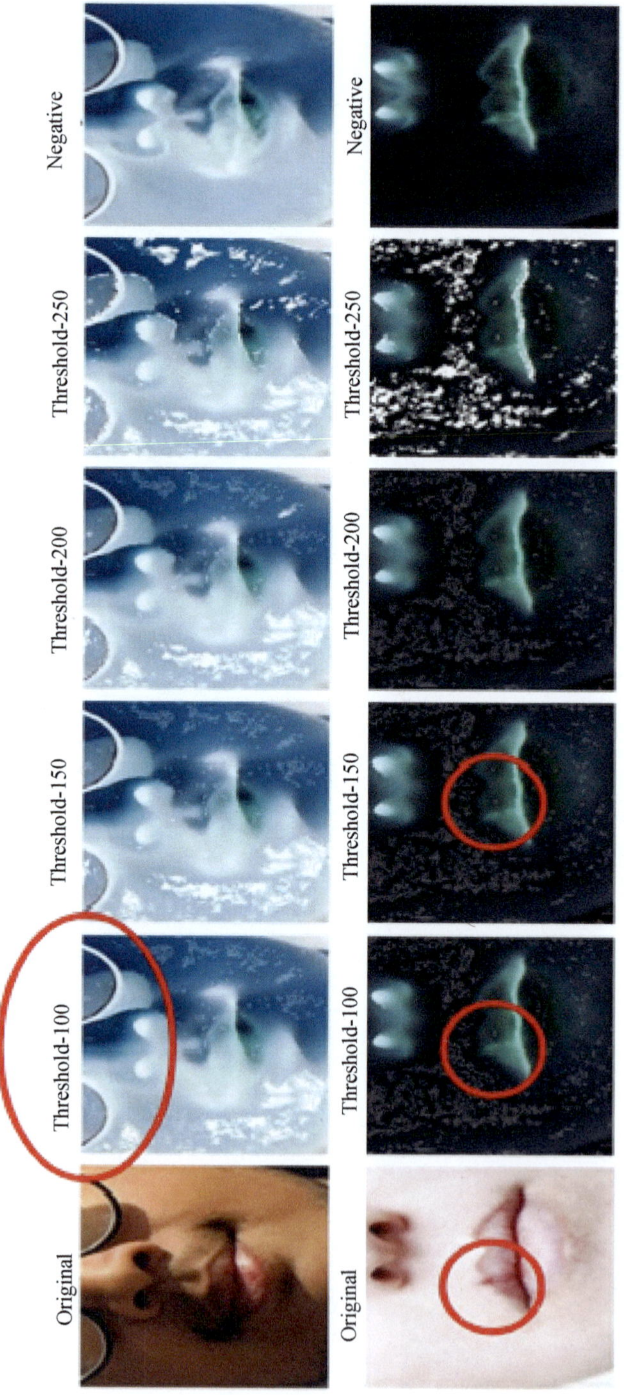

Fig. 6.13   Image of oral cancer

Conclusion

In this paper, a cancer cell detection and classification approach has been proposed based on convolutional neural networks (CNNs). The image datasets are also fed into the suggested model to obtain deep-learned characteristics. The CNN and ANN model is implemented using transfer learning and fine tuning. Performance measures after applying the discussed models to all the 4 image sets have been compared in this study. From the comparative study it can be said that the proposed model with the correct hyper tuning of threshold parameters used for segmentation performs better than the other network-based deep learning models for the image sets of Brain MRI & Cervical Cancer. For these two datasets, the proposed model outperformed previous generic models because it is more dependent on pixel intensities and uses just one feature to categorize the pictures. One of the other variables was selecting high-quality images for the dataset. However, it failed for the Chest CT may be due to the image set, as it has lines and noises that degrade the picture quality, lowering the model's accuracy. Oral Cancer (Lips & Tongue) image set is colored with numerous characteristics to determine, which was a bias for the model in determining and classifying the pictures, resulting in lower accuracy than the other models.

References

Albawi S., Mohammed T.A. and Al-Zawi S. 2017, August. Understanding of a convolutional neural network. In 2017 *International Conference on Engineering and Technology* (ICET) (pp. 1–6). Ieee.

Barik R., Naskar M.N.B., Chowdhury S. and Pal S. 2021. Cancer detection using cellular automata-based segmentation techniques. In 2021 Asian Conference on Innovation in Technology (ASIANCON) (pp. 1–6). IEEE.

Barik R., Nazma M., Naskar B.J. and Mallik S. 2021a. COVID-19 Detection System Using Cellular Automata-Based Segmentation Techniques. *Computational Intelligence and Healthcare Informatics*, pp. 313–23.

Brain tumor. (2022, February 23). Kaggle. https://www.kaggle.com/datasets/samudraneelbanerjee/brain-tumor

Cervical Cancer largest dataset (SipakMed). (2021, March 12). Kaggle. https://www.kaggle.com/datasets/prahladmehandiratta/cervical-cancer-largest-dataset-sipakmed

Chest CT-Scan images Dataset. (2020, August 20). Kaggle. https://www.kaggle.com/datasets/mohamedhanyyy/chest-ctscan-images

Gonzalez R.C. and Woods, R.E. (2002). Digital Image Processing. Prentice Hall, 2nd ed.

He K., Zhang X., Ren S. and Sun J. (2016). Deep residual learning for image recognition. *In proceedings of the IEEE conference on computer vision and pattern recognition* (pp. 770–78).

Kari J. (2013). Cellular Automata. Spring 2013.

Kwak N. (2016). Introduction to Convolutional Neural Networks (CNNs). LAMDA Group, China.

Oral Cancer (Lips and Tongue) images. (2020, October 6). Kaggle. https://www.kaggle.com/datasets/shivam17299/oral-cancer-lips-and-tongue-images

Senthil Kumar K., Venkatalakshmi K. and Karthikeyan K. 2019. Lung cancer detection using image segmentation by means of various evolutionary algorithms. *Computational and mathematical methods in medicine*, 2019. https://doi.org/10.1155/2019/4909846.

Simonyan K. and Zisserman A. (2014). Very deep convolutional networks for large-scale image recognition. *arXiv preprint arXiv:1409.1556.*

Szegedy C., Vanhoucke V., Ioffe S., Shlens J. and Wojna Z. (2016). Rethinking the inception architecture for computer vision. In *Proceedings of the IEEE conference on computer vision and pattern recognition* (pp. 2818–26).

7

Convolutional Neural Networks and Transfer Learning for Medical Image Analysis: A Comprehensive Review

Vinay Dubey,[1] Aakansha Gupta[1] and Rahul Katarya[1]*

Medical image analysis is vital in modern healthcare, helping to diagnose and cure a variety of disorders. Machine learning algorithms have resulted in significant advances in medical imaging, which are essential for disease detection and treatment planning. Convolutional Neural Network (CNN) is a powerful tool for medical imaging diagnostic help. Recent years have seen significant progress in the use of CNN and Transfer Learning (TL) techniques for medical imaging . This chapter presents an in-depth analysis of CNNs and transfer learning in medical imaging, highlighting their significant contributions to disease detection and treatment planning. CNNs excel in tasks such as feature extraction, segmentation, and classification, addressing challenges related to data scarcity and computational limitations. The study emphasizes the benefits of CNN and transfer learning, including increased accuracy and reduced resource needs, while acknowledging challenges such as interpretability and dataset diversity. The study emphasizes the effectiveness of CNNs in medical image classification tasks. It emphasizes the necessity for greater study into improving CNN and transfer learning methods for medical imaging and provides potential future research directions.

[1] Delhi Technological University, (Formerly Delhi College of Engineering), New Delhi-India.
* Corresponding author: aakanshagupta.74@gmail.com

Introduction

Timely diagnosis of medical anomalies is critical for preventing loss of lives and reducing trauma from injuries or diseases. Diseases such as tuberculosis, tumors, lung diseases, diabetic retinopathy, glaucoma, and heart diseases require an understanding of images from modalities such as X-rays, PET scans, CT scans, MRIs, ultrasound scans or single photon emission CT scans. However, challenges such as the scarcity of human experts, fatigue, high consultation charges, and variability in anomaly shapes, locations, and structures exist. Intelligent image-understanding systems are increasingly necessary to support the precise diagnosis and interpretation of medical images.

In recent years, image understanding systems have progressed rapidly, utilizing machine learning (ML) and deep learning (DL) approaches such as random forests (RFs), decision tree learning, restricted Boltzmann machines (RBMs), clustering, support vector machines (SVMs) and k-means nearest neighbor (K-NN). Efficient machine learning relies on extracting discriminating features, which can be challenging in image-understanding applications. To tackle this challenge, intelligent machines capable of autonomously learning and extracting features have been developed. A significant success in this domain is the CNN model, renowned for its capability to automatically learn and extract crucial features for understanding medical images. CNN gained prominence in 2012 with AlexNet's (Krizhevsky et al., 2017) victory in the ImageNet challenge, demonstrating high accuracy and low error rates. CNN is widely used in natural language processing, image and signal processing, and data analytics. Notably, GoogleNet's use of CNN achieved 89% accuracy in detecting cancer, surpassing the 70% accuracy of human pathologists (Team et al., 2016).

Computer-aided diagnosis (CAD) is a vital research field in medical imaging that employs ML algorithms to analyze historical patient imaging data and create models for assessing current conditions (Chan et al., 2020). This aids clinicians in making rapid decisions, with common imaging modalities including X-rays, CTscans, MRIs, PET scans, and ultrasound scans. Medical image processing focuses on enhancing interpretability and involves categories such as segmentation, detection, classification, enhancement, registration, and localization (Ker et al., 2018). The evolution from low-level methods to machine learning, and subsequently to artificial neural networks (ANNs), has been driven by the expanding complexity and size of medical imaging data (Niyas et al., 2022). Deep learning, particularly CNN, has made medical image processing more automated. A CNN is a type of neural network developed to manage pixel values and improve image classification scalability by identifying patterns within images using linear mathematical principles. Traditional CNN architectures involve stacking convolutional layers, but modern approaches like Inception, ResNet, and DenseNet introduce innovative methods for more efficient learning (Dutta et al., 2020). CNNs can serve as feature extractors, converting raw pixel data into detailed numerical features and replacing traditional extractors. These features can be used in classifier networks or machine learning algorithms to classify data. However, concerns exist about using deep CNN architectures in the field of radiology, as demonstrated in 2014 when introducing noise to data led to misclassifications (Jogin et al., 2018). Additionally, the effectiveness of deep learning relies on large-scale, well-annotated radiology images, posing challenges in terms of cost and labor for database creation in the medical industry (Goodfellow et al., 2014).

The chapter emphasizes the central role of people's health in medical care and highlights the vast amount of available medical data. It stresses the importance of using this data wisely to benefit the medical industry (Cai et al., 2020). Medical images, crucial for diagnosis and treatment, are often examined by radiologists, who compile reports (Chopra et al., 2022). However, human interpretation faces challenges like subjectivity, variations among interpreters, and limited time, leading to missed findings and lengthy turnaround times. This hampers the potential for evidence-based, individualized healthcare. The article introduces Artificial Intelligence (AI) as a broad field applied in healthcare, among other sectors (Mutasa et al., 2021). Machine learning, a subset of AI, highlights the capacity to learn from data and make decisions with minimum human participation. DL techniques, especially in medical imaging, have gained attention, with CNN being a key component (Bhatt et al., 2021).

Motivation and Purpose

CNN have contributed much in the area of image understanding, CNN-based techniques are ranked first in numerous image understanding problems. CNN has become a powerful method for medical images interpretation (Menze et al., 2015). Furthermore, CNN-based models such as CheXNet have been utilized to classify 14 distinct chest diseases outperforming the average performance of human experts (Philips et al., 2020). Researchers have successfully employed CNNs for a variety of applications in medical image understanding, including tumor identification and classification as benign or malignant, as well as detection of images from optical coherence tomography for conditions such as blood cancer, chest diseases and eye diseases (Arevalo et al., 2016, Kermany et al., 2018).

CNNs have also gained importance in coronavirus disease-2019 (COVID-19) detection using CT scan images and chest X-rays. CNNs are becoming a prominent topic in reputable publications that have set aside special issues to address problems with deep learning models. The extensive research on CNNs demonstrates their usefulness and widespread use, but different research communities are working on these applications at the same time, and the results of their dissemination are dispersed across a wide range of conference proceedings and journals.

Convolutional Neural Network

A CNN is a supervised deep-learning system that can distinguish one form of data from another. After taking images as input, it applies filters to convert the pixels into features. This structure consists of three general levels: the fully connected layer, the pooling layer, and the convolutional layer. The convolutional layer is the first layer in the CNN, while the fully connected layer comes last, followed by other convolutional or pooling layers. The convolutional block extracts visual features for the network to inspect and extract hidden correlations. Pooling layers are used to minimize the quantity of convolved features, also known as downsampling (Yadav and Jadav. 2019). Convolutional layers use the rectified linear unit (ReLu) function to stimulate neurons, whereas fully connected layers categorize inputs using a softmax activation function (Kiranyaz et al., 2016).

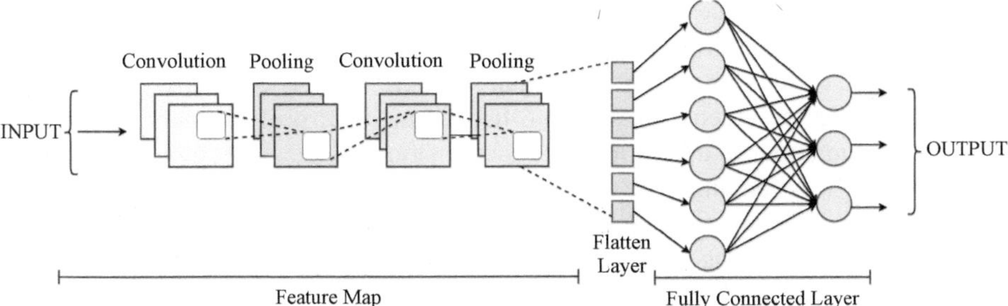

Fig. 7.1   Architecture of convolutional neural network

Figure 7.1 provides an in-depth description of the basic structure and characteristics of a CNN, which comprises the following components:

- **Convolutional Layer:** This is the initial layer of a CNN. It applies a set of reusable filters, referred to as kernels, to the input image to perform convolution operations. Specific features such as, textures, edges and forms in the input are detected by each filter. The layer's output is a set of feature maps that represent these features' location throughout the image. Certain variables, including stride and padding, may cause the feature maps to shrink in size.

- **Activation Function:** Following the convolution process, element-wise non-linearity is often introduced by using an activation function such as ReLU, which aids in the network's ability to learn increasingly intricate patterns.

- **Pooling Layer (or Subsampling Layer):** This layer performs a downsampling of the feature maps obtained from the convolutional layers. Average pooling and max pooling are widely used methods to decrease the spatial dimensions for feature maps while maintaining the most significant information. This helps in managing overfitting and lowers computing complexity.

- **Fully Connected Layer:** A fully connected layer or layers often come after several convolutional and pooling layers in a network. Classification and regression tasks are performed by these layers, which resemble those in a conventional neural net. They map the previously extracted features from the earlier levels to the appropriate class of output or values.

- **Flattening:** Before being passed to the fully connected layers from the convolutional/pooling layers, the data is flattened. The multi-dimensional feature maps are converted throughout this step into a one-dimensional vector that can be used in the fully connected layers.
- **Output Layer:** Based on the requirement, the final layer of the network offers predictions or outputs, such as probabilities of classes for classification and values in numbers for regression.

Medical Image Understanding

Medical imaging is necessary to see within organs and spot structural or functional abnormalities. Technologies such as ultrasound scanners, X-rays, MRI scans, PET scans, and CT scans record internal organ structure or function, displaying results as still images or videos. In the past, trained medical professionals used their skills and judgment to determine the exact position, dimensions, and shape of an abnormality (Sarvamangala et al., 2021).

Smart healthcare systems strive to achieve these objectives by leveraging intelligent medical image understanding. In medical image interpretation, the most crucial tasks are classification, segmentation, detection, and localization (Rana and Bhusan 2022).

Medical Image Classification

Medical image classification involves analyzing images from various diagnostic tests, such as CT scans, MRI scans, and X-rays, using ML techniques. The process of medical image classification includes selecting and labeling images from a predetermined set. Finding features in the image and applying those features to assign labels are the tasks involved in this assignment. Let L represent a pixel-based image, and $L1, L2,..., Lr$ represents the labels.

For every pixel x, a feature vector ξ, determining the value of ($f(x_i)$) obtained from the neighborhood $N(\chi)$ by 1, where,

$$x_i \in (f(x_0), f(x_1), f(x_2) \ldots \ldots \ldots \ldots f(x_k)) \qquad \ldots(1)$$

$$x_i \in N(\chi) \text{ for } i = 0, 1,... k.$$

A label is assigned to the image based on the list of labels $L1, L2,... Lr$.

Medical Image Segmentation

Medical image segmentation is the technique for segmenting medical images into significant pieces to detect features such as organs or anomalies. It facilitates the quantitative assessment of lesions or other anomalies, as well as understanding the image and extracting and recognizing features. The goal is to segment an image into parts with high correlations, which provides important data for pathological study and, as a result, diagnosis and treatment planning. Segmentation is the process of splitting an image into a finite set of areas.

Image L as a finite set of regions $R_1, R_1 \ldots \ldots \ldots R_s$ is expressed in Equation 2 as under:

$$L = \bigcup_{i=1}^{s} R_i, R_i \cap R_j = \varnothing \text{ and } i \neq j \qquad \qquad ...(2)$$

Medical Image Localization

Medical image localization involves recognizing and precisely designating certain locations or features of medical images, such as tumors or anomalies. The method entails collecting labeled data, processed images, utilizing techniques to pinpoint areas such as bounding boxes or landmark identification, training machine learning models, validating accuracy, refining the model, and using it in clinical practice. Image variability and the need for precisely labeled data are among the challenges faced with building precise localization models.

The localization function $f(I)$ on an image I calculates c, I_x, I_y, I_w, I_h, representing the class label, centroid x and y coordinates, and proportion of the bounding box to the image's width and height respectively as shown in equation 3.

$$f(I) = (c, I_x, I_y, I_w, I_h,) \qquad \qquad ...(3)$$

Medical Image Detection

The automatic identification of particular items or anomalies, such as tumors or fractures, within medical images is known as medical image detection. Using methods to find these objects such as object identification algorithms or deep learning, gathering labeled data, producing photos, training models, verifying the accuracy, improving the model, and incorporating it into clinical practice are all steps in the process. The unpredictability of images and the requirement for precisely labeled data to train accurate detection models present challenges.

Let I represent an image containing regions of interest or n objects. Then, the detection function (I) is calculates c, x_i, y_i, w_i, h_i which are the class label, centroid x, and y coordinates, and proportion of the bounding box to the width and height of the image, respectively as shown in equation 4.

$$\bigcup_{i=0}^{1} c, x_i, y_i, w_i, h_i = D(I) \qquad \qquad ...(4)$$

Evaluation Metrics for Image Understanding

The efficiency of medical images interpretation algorithms is evaluated by a variety of measures. The table used for calculating several assessment measures and showing algorithm performance is called the confusion matrix, sometimes referred to as the error matrix. It gives an understanding of the kinds of mistakes the classifier makes. Table 7.1. displays the confusion matrix of a binary classifier.

Here, correctly identified positives are indicated by True positives (TP), correctly identified negatives by True negatives (TN), wrongly identified positives by False positives (FP), and incorrectly identified negatives by False negatives (FN). FN is referred to as a miss, and FP is also known as a false error.

Table 7.1   Confusion matrix

Total test samples	*Predicted positive*	*Predicted negative*
Actual positive	TP	FN
Actual negative	FP	TN

The total of the right and wrong guesses is denoted by T and written as in equation 5.

$$T = T_p + T_N + F_P + F_N \qquad \qquad ...(5)$$

CNN on Medical Image Classification

In the last few years, the number of DL surveys has increased significantly. For example, a review of DL approaches used in pervasive sensing, bioinformatics and medical imaging has been presented which provides a comprehensive evaluation of DL algorithms for brain segmentation using MRI data (Ravi et al., 2017; Akkus et al., 2017). Another study highlights the achievements and drawbacks of DL techniques for medical image segmentation in this overview (Hesamian et al., 2019). Although the literature contains numerous survey studies, the majority of them focus on DL models such as recurrent neural networks (RNN), CNN, generative adversarial networks (GAN), or a specific application. Furthermore, there has been minimal discussion on the utility of CNN in the early detection of COVID-19.

While deep networks can extract features more precisely, they are computationally demanding. For this reason, Badža and Barjaktarović demonstrated a CNN architecture that accurately classified colorectal cancer histopathology images with a 22.7% error rate (Badža and Barjaktarović. 2020). They included five convolutional blocks, each with a dropout layer, to prevent overfitting. The model used 10-fold cross-validation to analyze 3064 MRI images and reached the highest accuracy of 95.56%.

The DL architecture used for segmenting images consists of an encoder and a decoder. The final output, which is typically a segmentation mask with the object's shape, is produced by the decoder after the encoder has used filters to extract information from the image. A fully convolutional network is an encoder-decoder model that uses 1×1 convolutions instead of dense layers to simulate fully connected layers (Shelhamer et al., 2017). Sun et al. designed a three-dimensional FCNN-based model for the multimodal segmentation of brain tumor images (Sun et al., 2021). The encoder included four paths for extracting multiscale picture characteristics. The four feature maps were concatenated and supplied into the decoder, and the model was used to segment the dataset using Dice following experimental validation on the 2019 Brain Tumor Segmentation Challenge dataset.

Mask regional CNN is another CNN variation that's utilized for segmenting medical images. Mask R-CNN is a two-stage object identification and segmentation architecture in which the region proposal network produces potential bounding boxes, and the second step constructs the segmentation mask from each box (He et al., 2020). A hybrid model that combines mask R-CNN and U-Net for pancreatic segmentation from CT images divides the system into two parts: Pancreas identification and pancreas segmentation. In pancreas localization, the region proposal network was used in conjunction with the mask production network to determine the bounding boxes of the pancreas portion, and the sub-region centered by the rough pancreas region was sliced (Dogan et al., 2021). Another paper proposed smaller image patches to reduce spatial information loss as well as variable attenuation ranges to improve visibility (Gao et al., 2016). The proposed CNN model used three lung attenuation ranges for the RGB images: Lower, normal, and higher. Jitter and cropping were used to improve the images in order to reduce overfitting. A basic Alexnet model incorporating the previously specified modifications was created, and its performance was compared to current CNN models that operate on picture patches.

ResNet and InceptionNet CNN models were also proposed, which demonstrated the efficacy of TL models with a test accuracy of 93%. One of the initial models proposed for COVID-19 detection was a rudimentary pre-trained AlexNet model developed and fine-tuned using chest X-ray images (Maghdid et al., 2020). The results were highly encouraging, with an accuracy of approximately 95% in distinguishing positive and negative patients.

Bassi and Attux proposed a DenseNet model trained twice using the transfer learning approach (Bassi and Attux. 2021) The image dataset was used to train the denseNet201 model, followed by the chest X-ray 14 dataset and the COVID-19 dataset. Tests were conducted on several combinations of training models initially using single TL, twice TL, and twice TL with output neuron retention. A proposal for an automated hyperparameter tuning inception-v4 (HPTI-v4) model for DR in color fundus image classification and detection was made in (Shankar et al., 2020). The images were segmented using a histogram-based model after being preprocessed with CLAHE to increase the contrast level. The Bayesian optimization method is used to tune hyperparameters, creating a probabilistic model based on previous validation results. The MESSIDOR DR dataset was utilized for classification, and the CNN model performed well, with 98.83% sensitivity, 99.68% specificity, and 99.49% accuracy. It was proposed that extensive augmentation and fine-tuning can overcome a lack of training data by segmenting tumor regions from an MR image using input-cascaded CNN, extensive augmentation, and then fine-tuning using data augmentation (Sajjad et al., 2019). The performance was compared to state-of-the-art methods, yielding a specificity, sensitivity, and accuracy of 96.58%, 88.41%, and 94.58%, respectively. In recent times, researchers have employed convolutional neural network-based models to extract distinctive and valuable features for the diagnosis of a variety of diseases, such as breast cancer, brain cancer, Parkinson's disease, heart disease, COVID-19 and Alzheimer's disease (AD) from medical images (Khvostikov et al., 2018). Previous research has demonstrated that these models yield a high degree of accuracy when compared to volumetric techniques that require manual physician interpretation and traditional machine learning. In a study the authors classified AD patients using a CNN model based on diffusion-tensor imaging and MRI (Liu et al., 2022). They found that when larger ROIs are used in conjunction with CNN architecture, classification performance shows that ROI size is not significant. The researchers employed a six-layered CNN, a 48 × 48 × 48 ROI, and a data fusion model to achieve 96.7% accuracy with AD-Normal Control in their case.

Ajagbe S.A. et al. used MRI scans to report on the use of deep convolutional neural networks and transfer learning models (VGG-16 and VGG-19) for AD diagnosis (Ajagbe et al., 2021). On the other hand, VGG-16 performed best in one of the six performance metrics (AUC), VGG-19 in three, and CNN in two (Recall, computational time, precision, F-1 score, accuracy, and AUC). The study's drawbacks included high computing power and the lack of a self-created dataset.

Pablo Villa-Pulgarin, J. et al. focused on classifying skin lesion cancers using CNN-based models DensNet-201, Inception-ResNet-V2, and Inception-V3 (Pablo et al., 2022). They examined the models using various workflows, data augmentation, and fine-tuning the optimization. The HAM10000 dataset produced the best results for their model, with an accuracy of 93% using the optimized DenseNet-201 model and 98% using the data augmentation stage. In another study, the predictive power of the transfer learning-based CNN models VGG-16, ResNet-50, and Inception-v3 was tested on a dataset of 233 MRIs (Srinivas et al., 2022). The models' accuracy was measured, and the results showed that the VGG-16 model performed significantly better than the other models with its trainable data. It utilizes 2 × 2 max-pool kernels and 3 × 3 convolution kernels with 138 million hyperparameters, resulting in a 44.9 percent decrease. This led to an increase in learning rates and a decrease in overfitting.CNN is a significant feature extractor; thus, employing it to identify medical images can avoid expensive and complicated feature engineering. Training an adequate model with small amounts of data is challenging, which is why CNN transfer learning is widely used in medical image classification tasks.

InceptionV3 was used with ImageNet-trained weight and TL on a dataset of more than one lakh optical coherence tomography images (Kermany et al., 2018). The CNN-based system outperformed six human experts in terms of specificity and sensitivity, resulting in an average accuracy, sensitivity, and specificity of 96.6%, 97.8%, and 97.4%, respectively. The researchers additionally verified their approach using a small pneumonia dataset including approximately 5,000 images, achieving a sensitivity of 93.2%, an average accuracy of 92.8%, and a specificity of 90.1%. This approach may finally assist in the rapid diagnosis of patients, resulting in earlier treatment and a higher cure rate. Furthermore, a study was conducted on how to use transfer learning to build an X-ray image classification system, which is a critical component of a computer-aided diagnosis system (Vianna. 2018). In comparison to two other models—training from scratch and a transfer learning model with simply a retrained final classification layer—the authors discovered that a fine-tuned transfer learning system with data augmentation efficiently alleviates overfitting and produces superior results (Raj et al., 2022).

Overall, our findings emphasize the importance of TL and CNNs in medical imaging diagnosis. Transfer learning is a useful technique to enhance the performance of CNN models that have already been trained for medical image analysis. CNNs are highly accurate and reliable in recognizing and classifying medical problems from images. Transfer learning reduces the quantity of data and computation needed for high accuracy by effectively applying knowledge from previously trained models to new tasks.

Although these approaches have resulted in promising results in the healthcare field, there remain some issues and constraints:

- One of the primary challenges in the application of TL and CNNs in medical imaging is the deficiency of diverse and extensive training datasets. Transfer learning approaches, like CNNs, primarily rely on large, diverse datasets to identify significant patterns. Thus, utilizing TL to CNNs can drastically minimize the resources and time required to train a CNN from the start while also improving the network's performance on the objective task.
- While CNNs demonstrate remarkable accuracy and reliability in medical image classification, the interpretability of learned features remains a challenge. Acknowledging that the complex representations learned by CNNs may present difficulties for medical professionals in understanding the underlying decision-making process, thus highlighting the "black box" nature of CNNs.
- Another pertinent issue is the scarcity of annotated medical imaging data, which is essential for training accurate and robust CNN models. This scarcity poses a significant constraint, particularly in specialized medical imaging applications where expert annotation is labor-intensive and time-consuming.

CNN Applications in Medical Image Classification

The appropriate categorization of medical images is critical to supporting medical treatment and therapy. For instance, an X-ray is the most effective method of diagnosing pneumonia (Cai et al., 2020). However, the diagnosis of pneumonia from chest X-rays requires the expertise of professional radiologists, who are in short supply and can be costly in certain areas (Zhou et al., 2021). Traditional machine learning techniques, such as SVMs, have long been used in the classification of medical images. Nevertheless, these approaches have the following drawbacks: Their development has been rather gradual in recent years, and their performance is well below the practical norm. Furthermore, the process of extracting and selecting features takes a lot of time and varies depending on the item (Dubey and Katarya. 2020). Deep neural networks (DNNs), particularly CNNs, have demonstrated notable performances and are extensively employed in changing image classification applications (Rawat and Wang. 2017). This section intends to provide an extensive review of Convolutional Neural Network applications in medical image classification. The ultimate aim is to encourage experts investigating medical image understanding to deploy convolutional neural networks in research and diagnostics.CNN has outperformed humans in medical image classification research. CheXNet, a 121-layer CNN trained on a dataset of over 100,000 frontal-view chest X-rays (Chest X-ray 14), outperformed four radiologists (Kermany et al., 2018).

Breast Tumors

One of the most prevalent types of cancer among women worldwide is breast cancer. It can be discovered with mammograms. To avoid mistakes, it is recommended that two radiologists read the same mammogram independently. CNNs serve an important role in brain tumor image classification due to their capacity to understand detailed patterns from MRI data. These models are trained to identify tumor-related attributes using convolutional, pooling, and fully connected layers after gathering and preprocessing data from brain tumor images. Evaluation criteria such as accuracy and precision assess the model's performance, which can be improved using fine-tuning and transfer learning approaches.

Heart Diseases

Using CNNs for heart disease diagnosis entails collecting and preprocessing medical data, such as X-ray or MRI scans, before developing and training CNN architecture to determine whether a patient has a heart issue. An electrocardiogram (ECG) assesses the electrical activity of the heart and detects irregularities. Transfer learning, normalization, and hyperparameter adjustment are used to improve the model's performance (Rustam et al., 2022).

Brain Tumors

Detecting brain tumors using CNNs requires acquiring a dataset of brain MRI scans with tumors and non-tumors, partitioning them into validation, training, and testing sets, and preprocessing the images. MRI scans provide detailed images of the brain for tumor diagnosis. Automatically segmenting a brain tumor requires high-level feature extraction, making it a difficult task (Özkaraca et al., 2023).

Coronavirus Disease-2019

COVID-19 is a pandemic disease that has quickly spread worldwide. RT-PCR is a routinely used diagnostic tool to diagnose COVID-19 infection. The gold standard for Coronavirus disease testing is RT-PCR. This is a labor-intensive, time-consuming, and complicated procedure with limited availability and low accuracy. In areas with limited access to RT-PCR kits, chest X-rays can be used for initial screening of COVID-19 and provide a more accurate diagnosis (Gupta and Katarya 2021, 2022, 2023).

Deep learning has been utilized by researchers to distinguish between COVID-19 and other causes of chest infections.

Immune Response Abnormalities

Detecting immune response problems with CNNs requires gathering and preparing different data, such as microscope pictures or assay results. Autoimmune illnesses occur when the immune system responds abnormally to a normal body part. In certain disorders, the immune system targets healthy cells. IIF on human epithelial-2 cells is used to detect autoimmune diseases. Identifying these patterns manually can take time (Bayramoglu et al., 2015).

Lung Diseases

Interstitial lung disease (ILD) causes scarring in the lung parenchyma, leading to respiratory difficulties. High-resolution computed tomography (HRCT) imagery distinguishes distinct forms of ILDs. HRCT pictures exhibit significant visual variance among classes and considerable visual resemblance within a single class. Accurate classification is tough. An approach was presented for the automatic classification of peri-fissural tumors (Ciompi et al., 2015). The authors approached the classification challenge through supervised learning and an ensemble of classifiers. Using OverFeat followed by Random Forest improved performance significantly. Using the Random Forest bagging technique improved the model performance. The proposed model achieved an AUC of 86.8%.

In medical image categorization, small kernel CNNs are CNN architectures that predominantly use small filter sizes in the convolutional layers. Smaller filters, such as 3×3 or 5×5, enable the network to detect fine details and patterns in images. According to a study using low-level textual information and non-linear activations improves classification performance (Anthimopoulos et al., 2016). The authors reduced the kernel size to 2×2 to include additional nonlinear activations. Smaller receptive fields were used to capture lower-level textual information.

Medical Image Classification using CNN

This study deals with using CNNs to analyze chest X-ray images to identify cases of pneumonia and non-pneumonia. The dataset is divided into training and test sets, including CNNs chosen for their performance in classification tasks. Throughout training, the model learns patterns that predict pneumonia from the training data. The test set is used to determine how well the model can generalize to new, previously unknown data. The ultimate goal is to use CNN techniques as a diagnostic tool, assisting in the automatic and efficient identification of pneumonia in chest X-ray scans and therefore contributing to enhanced medical diagnostics.

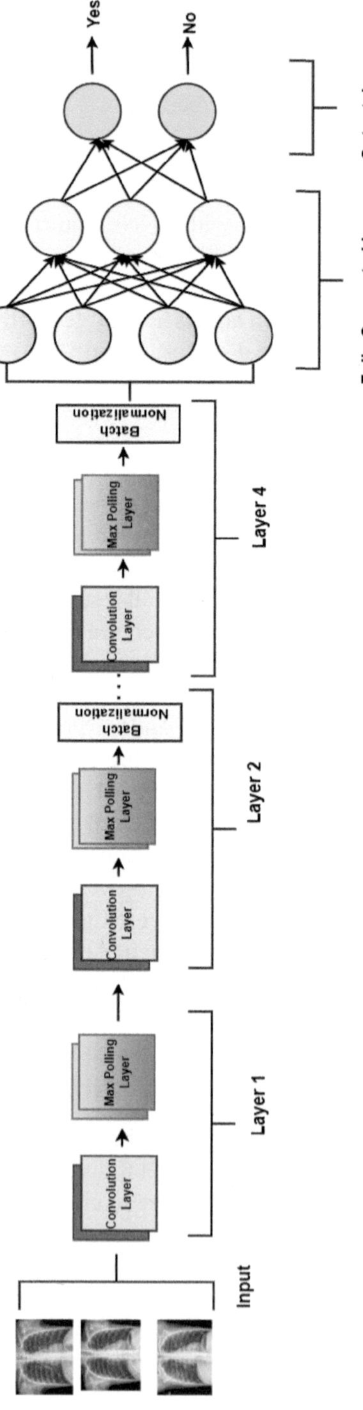

Fig. 7.2   CNN architecture for X-Ray image classifcation

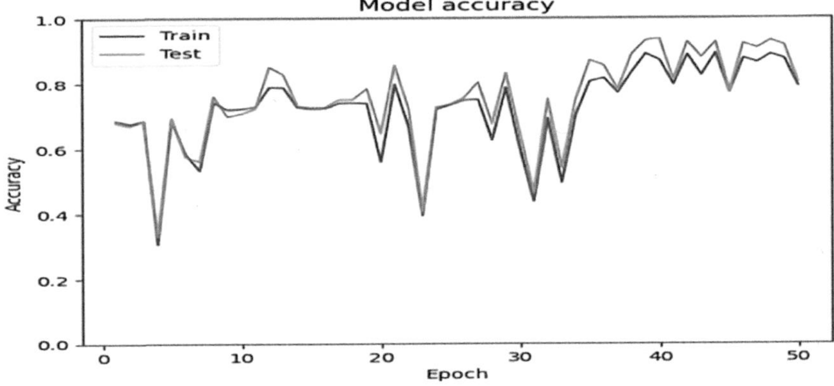

Fig. 7.3   Accuracy graph of CNN model

We presented a CNN model for binary image categorization in Figure 7.2. The model is made up of several convolutional blocks that have different filters and dropout rates. In some blocks, batch normalization is used, and the architecture comprises completely connected layers. To improve performance and reduce overfitting, CNN uses separable convolutions, batch normalization, dropout, and learning rate scheduling.

Figure 7.3 depicts the efficiency of the CNN model on both training and test datasets. On the test dataset, the model achieves a commendable 91% accuracy, demonstrating its usefulness. The X-axis on the graph reflects the number of epochs, whereas the Y-axis represents the accuracy scores.

Conclusion

Medical abnormalities vary in shape, size, appearance, location, and symptoms, complicating diagnosis and prognosis. Traditional ways to utilize human specialists require tiredness, oversight, high costs, and limited availability. ML-based healthcare systems require effective feature extraction strategies. CNN is a well-known and effective technique for extracting and learning low, mid, and high-level discriminatory characteristics from an input medical image, making it an excellent choice for resolving medical image interpretation challenges. This chapter shows that researchers have concentrated their efforts on the use of CNN to solve a variety of difficulties in medical image understanding. In terms of accuracy, sensitivity, AUC, DSC, time consumed, and so on, the CNN methods presented in this chapter were shown to outperform or complement existing classical and machine-learning methodologies. Because of the importance of the classification of medical images and the special problem of the small medical images' dataset, this work was chosen to research and assess the effectiveness of CNN-based classification on small chest X-ray datasets. Through our experiments, we discovered that CNN is the most successful approach for image classification.

References

Ajagbe S.A., Amuda K.A., Oladipupo M.A., AFE O.F. and Okesola K.I. et al., 2021. Multi-Classification of Alzheimer Disease on Magnetic Resonance Images (MRI) Using Deep Convolutional Neural Network (DCNN) Approaches. *International Journal of Advanced Computer Research* 11, no. 53 (March 31): 51–60.

Akkus Z., Galimzianova A., Hoogi A., Rubin D.L. and Erickson B.J. et al., 2017. Deep Learning for Brain MRI Segmentation: State of the Art and Future Directions. *Journal of Digital Imaging* 30, no. 4 (June 2): 449–59.

Anthimopoulos M., Christodoulidis S., Ebner L., Christe A. and Mougiakakou S. et al. 2016. Lung Pattern Classification for Interstitial Lung Diseases Using a Deep Convolutional Neural Network. *IEEE Transactions on Medical Imaging* 35, no. 5 (May): 1207–16.

Arevalo J., González F.A., Ramos-Pollán R., Oliveira J.L. and Guevara Lopez M.A. et al., 2016. Representation Learning for Mammography Mass Lesion Classification with Convolutional Neural Networks. *Computer Methods and Programs in Biomedicine* 127 (April): 248–57.

Badža M.M. and Barjaktarović M. 2020. Classification of Brain Tumors from MRI Images Using a Convolutional Neural Network. *Applied Sciences* 10, no. 6 (March 15): 1999.

Bassi P.R. and Attux R. 2021. A Deep Convolutional Neural Network for COVID-19 Detection Using Chest x-Rays. *Research on Biomedical Engineering* 38, no. 1 (April 2): 139–48.

Bayramoglu N., Kannala J. and Heikkila J. 2015. Human Epithelial Type 2 Cell Classification with Convolutional Neural Networks. *2015 IEEE 15th International Conference on Bioinformatics and Bioengineering (BIBE)* (November).

Bhatt D., Patel C., Talsania H., Patel J., Vaghela R. et al., 2021. CNN Variants for Computer Vision: History, Architecture, Application, Challenges and Future Scope. *Electronics* 10, no. 20 (October 11): 2470.

Cai L., Gao J. and Zhao D. 2020. A Review of the Application of Deep Learning in Medical Image Classification and Segmentation. *Annals of Translational Medicine* 8, no. 11 (June): 713–713.

Chan H., Hadjiiski L.M. and R.K. Samala. 2020. Computer-aided Diagnosis in the Era of Deep Learning. *Medical Physics* 47, no. 5 (May).

Chopra P., Junath N., Singh S.K., Khan S., Sugumar R. et al., 2022. Cyclic GAN Model to Classify Breast Cancer Data for Pathological Healthcare Task. *BioMed Research International* 2022 (July 21): 1–12.

Ciompi F., de Hoop B., van Riel S.J., Chung K., Th. Scholten E., Oudkerk M. et al., 2015. Automatic Classification of Pulmonary Peri-Fissural Nodules in Computed Tomography Using an Ensemble of 2D Views and a Convolutional Neural Network out-of-the-Box. *Medical Image Analysis* 26, no. 1 (December): 195–202.

Dogan R.O., Dogan H., Bayrak C. and Kayikcioglu T. 2021. A Two-Phase Approach Using Mask R-CNN and 3D U-Net for High-Accuracy Automatic Segmentation of Pancreas in CT Imaging. *Computer Methods and Programs in Biomedicine* 207 (August): 106141.

Dubey V. and Katarya, R. 2020. An Analysis of Machine Learning Techniques for Flood Mitigation. *Advances in Intelligent Systems and Computing* (July 31): 299–307.

Dutta P., Upadhyay P., De M. and Khalkar R.G. 2020. Medical Image Analysis Using Deep Convolutional Neural Networks: CNN Architectures and Transfer Learning. 2020. *International Conference on Inventive Computation Technologies* (ICICT) (February).

Gao M., Bagci U., Lu L., Wu A., Buty M. et al., 2018. Holistic Classification of CT Attenuation Patterns for Interstitial Lung Diseases via Deep Convolutional Neural Networks. Computer Methods in Biomechanics and Biomedical Engineering: Imaging & amp; *Visualization* 6, no. 1 (June 6): 1–6.

Goodfellow Ian, Shlens Jonathon and Szegedy Christian. 2014. Explaining and Harnessing Adversarial Examples. arXiv 1412.6572.

Gupta A. and Katarya R. 2022. Possibility of the COVID-19 Third Wave in India: Mapping from Second Wave to Third Wave. *Indian Journal of Physics* 97, no. 2 (July 14): 389–99.

Gupta A. and Katarya R. 2023. A Deep-SIQRV Epidemic Model for COVID-19 to Access the Impact of Prevention and Control Measures. *Computational Biology and Chemistry* 107 (December): 107941.

Gupta A. and Katarya R. 2021. PAN-LDA: A Latent Dirichlet Allocation Based Novel Feature Extraction Model for COVID-19 Data Using Machine Learning. *Computers in Biology and Medicine* 138 (November): 104920.

He K., Gkioxari G., Dollar P. and Girshick R. 2020. Mask R-CNN. IEEE Transactions on Pattern *Analysis and Machine Intelligence* 42, no. 2 (February 1): 386–97.

Hesamian M.H., Jia W., He X. and Kennedy P. 2019. Deep Learning Techniques for Medical Image Segmentation: Achievements and Challenges. *Journal of Digital Imaging* 32, no. 4 (May 29): 582–96.

Jogin M., Mohana, M.S., G.D. Madhulika, R.K. Divya, Meghana et al., 2018. Feature Extraction Using Convolution Neural Networks (CNN) and Deep Learning. 2018 3rd IEEE International Conference on Recent Trends in Electronics, Information & amp; *Communication Technology* (RTEICT) (May).

Ker J., Wang L., Rao J. and Lim T. 2018. Deep Learning Applications in Medical Image Analysis. *IEEE Access* 6: 9375–89.

Kermany D.S., Goldbaum M., Cai W., Valentim C.C., Liang H. et al., 2018. Identifying Medical Diagnoses and Treatable Diseases by Image-Based Deep Learning. Cell 172, no. 5 (February).

Khvostikov A., Aderghal K., Benois-Pineau J., Krylov A. and Catheline G. et al., 2018. 3D CNN-based classification using sMRI and MD-DTI images for Alzheimer disease studies.

Kiranyaz S., Ince T. and Gabbouj M. 2016. Real-Time Patient-Specific ECG Classification by 1-D Convolutional Neural Networks. *IEEE Transactions on Biomedical Engineering* 63, no. 3 (March): 664–75.

Krizhevsky A., Sutskever I. and Hinton G.E. 2017. ImageNet Classification with Deep Convolutional Neural Networks. *Communications of the ACM* 60, no. 6 (May 24): 84–90.

Liu Z., Lu H., Pan X., Xu M., Lan R. et al., 2022. Diagnosis of Alzheimer's Disease via an Attention-Based Multi-Scale Convolutional Neural Network. *Knowledge-Based Systems* 238 (February): 107942.

Maghdid Halgurd & Asaad, Aras & Ghafoor et al., 2020. Diagnosing COVID-19 Pneumonia from X-Ray and CT Images using Deep Learning and Transfer Learning Algorithms.

Menze B.H., Jakab A., Bauer S., Kalpathy-Cramer J., Farahani K. et al., 2014. The Multimodal Brain Tumor Image Segmentation Benchmark (Brats). *IEEE Transactions on Medical Imaging* 34, no. 10 (October): 1993–2024.

Mutasa S., Sun S. and Ha R. 2021. Understanding Artificial Intelligence Based Radiology Studies: CNN Architecture. *Clinical Imaging* 80 (December): 72–76.

Niyas S., Pawan S.J. Anand Kumar M. and Rajan J. 2022. Medical Image Segmentation with 3d Convolutional Neural Networks: A Survey. *Neurocomputing* 493 (July): 397–413.

Özkaraca O., Bağrıaçık O.İ. Gürüler H., Khan F., Hussain J. et al., 2023. Multiple Brain Tumor Classification with Dense CNN Architecture Using Brain MRI Images. *Life* 13, no. 2 (January 28): 349.

Phillips N.A., Rajpurkar P., Sabini M., Krishnan R., Zhou S. et al., 2020. Chexphoto: 10,000+ photos and transformations of chest X-rays for benchmarking deep learning robustness, arXiv.org. Available at: https://arxiv.org/abs/2007.06199 (Accessed: 15 January 2024).

Raj H., Gupta A. and Katarya R. 2022. Extract It! Product Category Extraction by Transfer Learning. *Lecture Notes in Networks and Systems:* 95–105.

Rana M. and Bhushan M. 2022. Machine Learning and Deep Learning Approach for Medical Image Analysis: Diagnosis to Detection. *Multimedia Tools and Applications* 82, no. 17 (December 24): 26731–69.

Ravi D., Wong C. Deligianni F., Berthelot M., Andreu-Perez J. et al., 2017. Deep Learning for Health Informatics. *IEEE Journal of Biomedical and Health Informatics* 21, no. 1 (January): 4–21.

Rawat W. and Wang Z. 2017. Deep Convolutional Neural Networks for Image Classification: A Comprehensive Review. *Neural Computation* 29, no. 9 (September): 2352–2449.

Rustam F., Ishaq A., Munir K., Almutairi M., Aslam N. et al., 2022. Incorporating CNN Features for Optimizing Performance of Ensemble Classifier for Cardiovascular Disease Prediction. *Diagnostics* 12, no. 6 (June 15): 1474.

Sajjad M., Khan S., Muhammad K., Wu W., Ullah A. et al., 2019. Multi-Grade Brain Tumor Classification Using Deep CNN with Extensive Data Augmentation. *Journal of Computational Science* 30 (January): 174–82.

Sarvamangala D.R. and Kulkarni R.V. 2021. Convolutional Neural Networks in Medical Image Understanding: A Survey. *Evolutionary Intelligence* 15, no. 1 (January 3): 1–22.

Shankar K., Zhang Y., Liu Y., Wu L. and Chen C.H. 2020. Hyperparameter Tuning Deep Learning for Diabetic Retinopathy Fundus Image Classification. *IEEE Access* 8: 118164–118173.

Shelhamer E., Long J. and Darrell T. 2017. Fully Convolutional Networks for Semantic Segmentation. *IEEE Transactions on Pattern Analysis and Machine Intelligence* 39, no. 4 (April 1): 640–51.

Srinivas C., N.P.K.S., Zakariah M., Alothaibi Y.A., Shaukat K., Partibane B. et al., 2022. Deep Transfer Learning Approaches in Performance Analysis of Brain Tumor Classification Using MRI Images. *Journal of Healthcare Engineering* 2022 (March 8): 1–17.

Sun J., Peng Y., Guo Y. and Li D. 2021. Segmentation of the Multimodal Brain Tumor Image Used the Multi-Pathway Architecture Method Based on 3D FCN. *Neurocomputing* 423 (January): 34–45.

Team The & Al-Rfou, Rami and Alain, Guillaume & Almahair et al., 2016. *Theano: A Python framework for fast computation of mathematical expressions.*

Vianna V.P., 2018. Study and development of a Computer-Aided Diagnosis system for classification of chest x-ray images using convolutional neural networks pre-trained for ImageNet and data augmentation.

Villa-Pulgarin J.P., Ruales-Torres A.A., Arias-Garzon D., Bravo-Ortiz M.A., Arteaga-Arteaga, H.B. et al., 2022. Optimized Convolutional Neural Network Models for Skin Lesion Classification. Computers, Materials & amp; Continua 70, no. 2: 2131–48.

Yadav S.S. and Jadhav S.M. 2019. Deep Convolutional Neural Network Based Medical Image Classification for Disease Diagnosis. *Journal of Big Data* 6, no. 1 (December).

Zhou S.K., Greenspan H., Davatzikos C., Duncan J.S., Van Ginneken B. et al., 2021. A Review of Deep Learning in Medical Imaging: Imaging Traits, Technology Trends, Case Studies with Progress Highlights, and Future Promises. *Proceedings of the IEEE* 109, no. 5 (May): 820–38.

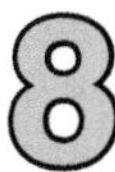

Multi-Objective Optimization Enabled Improved Feature Selection

Shreya,[1] Adarsh Kumar Arya,[1] Devanshi Srivastava[1] and Ashish Kapoor[1]*

Data mining and machine learning researchers have recently shown significant interest in feature selection. Feature selection is a well-studied subject in machine learning, aiming to identify the most effective characteristics that might enhance accuracy. Several studies have used particular methods and algorithms to choose numerous characteristics. This work aims to comprehensively analyze the problems and concerns associated with the multi-objective feature selection problem. Additionally, it seeks to evaluate and explore the many strategies presented to address this problem. The results of the analysis of this research indicate that a definitive solution to the issue of multi-objective feature selection has not yet been found. The authors anticipated that the presented review would serve as the primary repository of the strategies and methodologies used to address the issue of multi-objective feature selection. Moreover, ongoing obstacles and concerns are briefly discussed to identify potential areas of research that need futher investigation.

Introduction

Diverse problem domains often exhibit a variety of features in machine learning. Consequently, identifying an appropriate set of features while avoiding duplicates

[1] Department of Chemical Engineering, Harcourt Butler Technical University, Kanpur, India.
* Corresponding author: aarya@hbtu.ac.in

offers a considerable challenge. In dataset analysis, it has been discovered that characteristics demonstrate a lack of significance due to repetition and irrelevance within those attributes. As a result, it is crucial to emphasize that combining the mentioned features does not provide favorable results and often results in suboptimal classification accuracy. Thus, the primary objective of feature selection is to maximize the classification algorithm efficacy by choosing subsets of significant traits for a vast collection of potential candidates. The expulsion of unnecessary features decreases data dimensions, which lengthens the learning process by simplifying the generated model and improving performance (Guyon and Elisseeff). Because feature selection comes within the category of NP-hard problems, it presents a significant challenge. The task thoroughly analyzes a considerable search space with many $2n$ potential outcomes. The variable 'n' denotes the number of available attributes for investigation. The issue's complexity escalates considerably when the value of n increases due to developments in data-collection methods in all areas.

In contrast to feature selection, feature extraction procedures, such as 'Principal Component Analysis' (PCA) and 'Linear Discriminant Analysis' (LDA), generate new features by merging or changing existing features via a functional mapping (Wold et al., 1987; Balakrishnama et al., n.d). Therefore, the search space is constrained. Consequently, our assessment is restricted to methods for selecting qualities. To solve the problem of high dimensionality, the main objective of feature selection is to enhance classification performance by minimizing the number of features. Characteristic selection may be seen as a multi-objective problem aimed at achieving a balance between two conflicting aims. In recent years, research has made strides in developing multi-objective algorithms that use feature selection to overcome these issues, given the available tools and methodologies. This study assembles research papers from well-known databases and journals such as Web of Science', 'Science Direct', 'IEEE Xplore', 'Scopus', and others. Our research aims to conduct a comprehensive review of the most recent accomplishments in 'multi-objective feature selection', as well as to identify the obstacles and current issues that must be addressed in future research. This study aims to engage scholars interested in multi-objective optimization paradigms, encouraging them to develop practical approaches for addressing growing feature selection difficulties.

A Multi-Objective Optimization Approach to Feature Selection

'Multi-objective optimization', a core part of optimization, deals with complex issues involving many goals that are intrinsically in conflict with each other, necessitating their simultaneous optimization. In traditional optimization issues, it is expected to meet a single objective function that must be optimized while constrained by multiple constraints. It is critical to acknowledge the presence of numerous objective functions that need concurrent optimization in the 'Multi-Objective Optimization' arena. The existence of this quality automatically leads to the creation of trade-offs between the goals. The primary goal of 'Multi-Objective Optimization' (MOO) is to find a collection of optimum solutions in terms of all goals or, at the very least, not be susceptible to dominance. According to a study, the idea of dominance suggests a scarcity of alternative solutions that surpass the chosen strategy across all goal (Marler and Arora. 2004).

The formalization of a multi-objective issue may be formally expressed as follows:

'Minimize' (or 'maximize') $f(x) = f_1(x), f_2(x), \ldots, f_m(x)$ ...(1)

subject to $g(x) \leq 0, h(x) = 0$ ...(2)

The 'choice variables' are represented by the vector x, the ith 'objective function' is denoted by $f_i(x)$, the 'inequality constraints' are represented by $g(x)$, and the 'equality constraints' are represented by $h(x)$. A realizable solution is capable of meeting Equation (2). The concept of dominance is employed sometimes to compare two feasible solutions based on their objective function values (von Lücken et al., 2014). An evaluation is needed to evaluate the superiority of two possible solutions, x, and x's. Iff : x will be controlled by 'x'.

- For all objectives i in 1, 2,..., m, $f_i(x') \leq f_i(x)$ and there exists at least one objective j in 1, 2,..., m such that $f_j(x) \prec f_j(x)$

Simply put, a solution x' is said to dominate a solution x if it is equal to or better than x in all objectives and better than x in at least one. As a result, if any other alternative solution does not outperform solution x, it is said to be 'Pareto optimum' or 'non-dominated.' The Pareto front collects Pareto-optimal solutions that reflect the best trade-offs between the goals (Das et al., 2021).

MOO approaches are extensively utilized in various domains, including computer science, engineering, and economics. This is primarily due to their expertise in tackling complicated optimization problems with many goals. 'MOO algorithms' have been employed in 'recommender systems' to increase suggestion efficacy and customization (Concha-Carrasco et al., 2023).

MOO is a technique used in 'Recommender Systems' (RSs) to address the problem of focusing on a single goal and overlooking other important objectives like variety, innovation, and serendipity. Multi-Objective Recommender Systems (MORS) aims to deliver accurate, personalized suggestions that fit consumers' interests and requirements, improving user satisfaction, participation, and interactions with the recommender system. MORS uses approaches like 'Pareto optimization', 'constraint-based optimization', and 'weighted sum optimization' to create a balanced trade-off between multiple goals and deliver personalized suggestions. Implementing a model-based method maximizes attaining multiple goals, producing personalized and appropriate suggestions for each user. MOO approaches increase the efficiency of building and deploying a multi-objective optimization recommendation system.

Deterministic approaches are multi-objective optimization methods that use 'mathematical programming techniques', 'heuristic methods') and 'scalarization methods' (Chen et al., 2021; Vyas et al., 2022; Seymen et al., 2021). These methods solve optimization problems and determine the best solution using linear, non-linear, and integer programming. Scalarization approaches convert complex issues into singular problems by merging goals into a scalar target function, enabling conventional optimization techniques. Heuristic techniques use empirical methodology to uncover solutions in complex scenarios. However, these strategies may not be sufficient for complex optimization issues with multi-modality, discontinuity, and noisy landscapes. Objective functions with non-differentiability, non-continuity, nonlinearity, noise, flatness, multidimensionality, or multiple local minima are often encountered in real-world problems. Traditional optimization approaches often struggle to find the best solution for these issues, necessitating the use of more complex optimization techniques.

Over the past two decades, machine learning (MOO) Multi-objective optimization approaches have significantly improved and addressed complex optimization and search issues (Sharma and Kumar. 2022). Stochastic-based methods, such as swarm intelligence, evolutionary algorithms, and random search-based methods, have gained popularity as an alternative to deterministic approaches (Concha-Carrasco et al., 2023; Chai et al., 2020; Tran et al., 2022). These techniques are designed to solve complex problems with non-linear and non-convex objective functions. Evolutionary algorithms replicate the natural selection process, and have gained prominence as optimization and computational intelligence methods (Yani Xue et al., 2022). Swarm intelligence algorithms replicate the collective behavior of dispersed systems and contain self-organizing skills to find the best solution (Lu et al., 2020). Random search techniques produce solutions at random and evaluate them based on their fitness. Proper choice and configuration of stochastic techniques are crucial for optimizing complex issues while considering simulation processing needs.

Stochastic learning methods are a subset of MOO methodologies that extract information from data and solve optimization issues using stochastic processes. Two popular approaches are 'multi-objective reinforcement learning' (MORL) and 'multi-objective deep learning' (MODL) (Geng et al., 2023; Yıldırım et al., 2021). MORL focuses on developing optimum decision-making strategies in settings with multiple objectives using policy gradients, actor-critic frameworks, and value function approximation. MODL uses deep neural networks to understand the 'Pareto front' of MOO problems, beneficial for high-dimensional input fields. Stochastic learning techniques are popular in MOO research because they effectively solve complex and high-dimensional problems.

Feature Selection

Feature selection, a fundamental data preprocessing method, is pivotal in identifying a given dataset's salient, influential, and noteworthy attributes. The proposed methodology entails meticulously curating a subset comprising distinctive and pertinent features from various attributes. This subset is then employed to represent a given data record within a dataset effectively, thereby facilitating the process of modeling predictions (El-Kenawy et al., 2020). Figure 8.1 illustrates a general concept of feature selection, where a given feature set is subjected to a selection process.

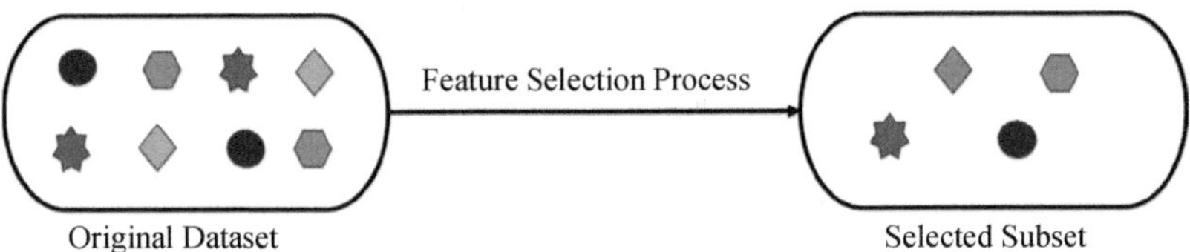

Fig. 8.1   Concept of feature selection

Finally, the most relevant or optimal feature sets are selected. 'Feature selection' is a method in feature engineering that aims to reduce the complexity of a job by using a particular attribute or item from a collection. This streamlines the process of categorization. The principal objective for the feature selection difficulties pertains to the reduction of dimensions within an extensive multi-dimensional dataset. Feature selection is a vital technique for efficiently extracting information from situations that include many attributes. The fundamental challenge of feature selection is to identify the optimal subset of features from a source dataset that may have many attributes. An arduous task arises when dealing with a large dataset, as extracting accurate correlations and arriving at a conclusive outcome becomes difficult. This challenge stems from the coexistence of pertinent and extraneous factors within the dataset. Selecting all the attributes would significantly influence the outcome. Therefore, to determine the best solution, it is crucial to choose the characteristics directly relevant to the current situation carefully.

Moreover, it is recommended to steer clear of factors that might influence the outcome, as they may lead to inaccurate results or hinder the progress of the research. Feature selection involves discovering and selecting the most impactful attributes from a dataset that substantially affect the desired prediction variable or outcome. This may be accomplished either by human or automated means. Including extraneous characteristics in the dataset may harm the precision of models and result in the model learning useless information. Therefore, a smaller portion of data is created from the original dataset to exclude irrelevant attributes. Attribute removal during the feature selection process may provide valuable insights into data size, reduce computation time and resource needs, lower dimensions, and improve the efficiency of the predictive model.

Prediction algorithms can uncover hidden intricacies in systems, enhancing operational efficiency. In COVID-19 management, timely detection is crucial due to the lack of widely recognized treatment options (Mansour et al., 2022). Key attributes for prognostication include symptoms like fever, headache, difficulty breathing, sore throat, coughing up phlegm, weakness, and muscle pain. Physical characteristics like weight, height, phone number, and address may not be relevant. Therefore, excluding this information during feature selection in disease-detecting simulations will enable prompt identification and containment of COVID-19. The primary goal is to reduce the number of attributes significantly.

Nevertheless, this reduction does not necessarily compromise the reliability of the model. Consequently, the effectiveness of the selection process is contingent upon two pivotal factors: 'enhancing the level of accuracy' and 'reducing the quantity of attributes'. The categorization of 'feature selection methods' is illustrated in Figure 8.2.

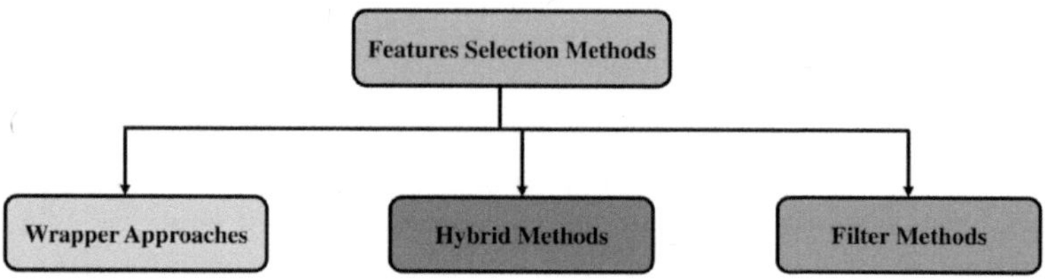

Fig. 8.2   Classification of feature selection methods

Filter Methods

'Filter techniques' generally have less processing overheads than wrapper alternatives. Filter approaches analyze data using specific criteria rather than learning algorithms. Explored places with lower-ranking criteria are purposely excluded. Two main filter algorithms are univariate and multivariate. A univariate system evaluates each property separately, whereas a multivariate technique evaluates all qualities simultaneously. Many research studies have used different assessment methods to improve feature subset selection. Methods include feature correlation, relief algorithm, mutual information, principal component analysis (PCA), and Fisher score (Gu et al., 2011). The absence of a learning system may hinder decision-making in these solutions. Metaheuristics that efficiently meet criteria may handle huge feature spaces, improving efficiency and the dragonfly algorithm (DA) search efficiency with ten chaotic maps (Sayed et al., 2018). They also determine the optimum features for quick convergence and recognizing dangerous compounds. After messy data processing, a 'support vector machine' was used. The experiment proved the 'Gauss chaotic map's' data processing superiority. Yu Xue et al. suggest using Relief scores to test biological trait discrimination to initialize the population in 'Particle Swarm Optimization' (PSO) (Yu Xue et al., 2019). They examined the difference between the sample and its similar and dissimilar neighbors. The threshold selection determines the number of characteristics (Renuka Devi and Sasikala. 2019). They used MapReduce to analyze large datasets, which required segmentation and parallel processing. BA reduces data dimensionality. After that, the ensemble approach uses a 'multi-layer perceptron artificial neural network classifier to find important traits. This method cuts processing time and improves accuracy. Additionally, it detects and assesses pre-existing and incoming feature drifts. The recommended 'multi-objective feature selection' strategy uses mutual knowledge and a genetic algorithm to evaluate solutions. The Genetic Algorithm (GA) evaluates solutions using merging, sorting, and crowding distance. In a study, for datasets of different sizes Emine and Yuker recommended using the social spider algorithm (SSA) to decrease the 'binary search space (Emine and Ülker. 2020).' The binary search space is assessed using S- and

V-shaped transfer functions. Each possible optimum solution becomes high-quality using a crossover strategy. BinSSA4 surpasses other algorithms in fitness, standard deviation, number of features, and accuracy when paired with a crossover operator. Peng and others recommended increasing network intrusion detection investigation to boost ACO performance. The recommended solution avoids local optimums by employing a well-built fitness function, pheromone mitigation, and encouraging particular methods (Peng et al., 2018).

Wrapper Approaches

Wrapper techniques involve determining feasible subsets of traits and assessing their significance, with the model repeating both stages until the termination condition is met. The wrapper-based feature selection algorithm finds solutions until it meets the accuracy rate goal or the fewest number of features. However, wrapper solutions have significant limits and cost more computationally than filtering. Extensive studies have explored wrapper-based feature selection for handling high-dimensional datasets. Techniques such as 'butterfly optimization algorithm' (BOA) (Arora and Anand. 2019), 'grasshopper optimization' method (Zakeri and Hokmabadi. 2019), 'ABC approach' (Rao et al., 2019), 'gradient boosting decision tree algorithm', 'max-min ant system' (MMAS) pheromone update rule mechanism (Montemayor and Crisostomo. 2019), S- and V-shaped dynamic behavior transfer functions (M.M. Mafarja et al., 2018), chaotic maps, wrapper-based KNN, and 'binary feature selection' (Sofiane and Zouache. 2019) have been used to improve classification accuracy while minimizing features.

The wrapper-based KNN integrates the calculated Euclidean distance, two rounds of the 'whale optimization algorithm' (WOA), 'evolutionary operators', and 'binary feature selection' techniques. The crossover and mutation WOA algorithm outperforms the 'GA', 'PSO', and 'ant lion optimizer approaches' (M.M. Mafarja and Mirjalili. 2018). A binary feature selection technique maximizes accuracy while decreasing features, and the 'discrete cosine transform' (DCT) with a fixed-size window technique is employed to understand data streaming's fundamental features (Aydoğdu and Ekinci. 2020). Auto-feature selection finds the best-performing subset and GWO and WOA improve the combination metaheuristic wrapper-based feature subset selection. Hybridization improves immature convergence and stagnation to local optima. The 'sine-cosine approach' to the exploration stage improves information quality, and the optimization technique is more accurate on 11 out of 16 datasets (Hussain et al., 2021). Using opposite point exploration and disruption is recommended to prevent feature over-randomization due to local CS algorithm optimization difficulties (Kelidari and Hamidzadeh. 2020). These aspects aid complex data exploration and selection, ultimately improve classification accuracy while minimizing features. The 'slime mold algorithm' (SMA) has been optimized using OBL to avoid premature convergence and sluggish movement (Wazery et al., 2021). Other studies have suggested early FPA population generation, chaotic maps for CS exploration, and two-population elite preservation techniques for cuckoo locations. Firefly and binary PSO have been combined for more accurate global search. Competitive Swarm Optimizer with KNN has been used for large-scale optimization problems. Li and others built an OBL mechanism that addresses engineering application problems, tracking variant convergence and balancing exploration and exploitation without fitness tests (Li et al., 2021). Rathasamuth and Pasupa identified swine breed categorization overfitting using feature selection and Binary FPA (Rathasamuth and Pasupa, 2019). Tan and his associates reduced three-dimensional feature spaces by pruning unnecessary features, using DE, GA, and PSO input. Multilingual spam detection using WOA and SVM is also discussed (Tan et al., 2020). Artificial fish swarm optimization with crossover operation categorizes text and boosts local search. FPA advises reducing unnecessary biological data and boosting population diversity and FPA algorithm search performance (Yan et al., 2019). Adaptive Gaussian mutation and absolute balancing group approach boost population diversity and FPA algorithm search performance, KNN measures classification accuracy, are outperforms cutting-edge techniques in experiments. Hybridization of 'Biogeography-Based Optimization' and 'Genetic Algorithm' for Breast Density Classification Hans and Kaur, combine methods from various fields (Hans and Kaur, 2021). Alsaleh and Binsaeedan employed ABC and CS to discover network issues with less characteristics (Alsaleh and Binsaeedan. 2021). Almazini and Ku-Mahamud presented intrusion detection swarm methods (Almazini and Ku-Mahamud. 2021). On the other hand Grey Wolf Optimization balanced exploration and exploitation to pick the finest traits. Overall, these studies have shown promising results in optimizing algorithms for various applications, including swine breed categorization, audio processing, and intrusion detection.

Hybrid Method

The mixed technique combines the most relevant aspects of numerous feature selection procedures, such as 'filter-wrapper'. The primary objective is to increase the solution's stability by merging well-known feature subset selection strategies. The resulting solutions will be radically different when dealing with a tiny dataset with many features and a small portion of the training data. By integrating specific attributes gained from other ways, the solutions become clearer, ensuring the quality of the selected qualities is maintained. Ghosh and his team presented a 'hybrid technique' incorporating a 'bio-inspired algorithm' in their investigation (Ghosh et al., 2019). To pick relevant characteristics, this method applies a filtering strategy. The wrapper approach then assesses the feature sets derived from their quality. Suggestions for improving feature selection have been posted, including an improved memory to keep the best ant and a consistent pheromone updating technique.

Metaheuristic Algorithms for Multiclass Feature Selection

In recent decades, feature selection problems have garnered significant attention from researchers, who have been exploring metaheuristic algorithms as a potential

Table 8.1   Lists a comparison between the techniques used for feature selection

Technique Types	*Feature selection*	*Feature Selection Methods' Functionality and Drawbacks*	*Disadvantages*
Semi-Supervised	Graph based	Clustering of original features into multiple dominating sets of dependent features and a limited set of features.	Not a good approximator. Multimodal image feature acquisition and division employ this approach.
	Co-Training based	Combines two key unlabelled traits to predict the exam.	It discovers irrelevant data and examines how surplus characteristics affect semi-supervised learning.
Supervised	Correlation based	A multivariate channel chooses uncorrelated feature subsets.	It indicates strong class ties.
	Lasso regularization	Contracting regression coefficients and reducing elements to zero regularizes model boundaries.	This approach requires the number of model boundary supreme characteristics rather than target labor.
Un-Supervised	Filer	Selects the most relevant features based on the information's characteristics without using grouping techniques to regulate the inquiry of significant elements.	This method has speed and flexibility issues.
	Wrapper	Grouping results are used to evaluate feature subsets. Determining feature subsets that increase grouping results was used to construct this strategy.	Unfortunately, feature selection approaches are computationally expensive and limited to a specific grouping strategy.
	Hybrid	Misuse of filter and wrapper properties.	It seeks a balance between proficiency (computational effort) and viability (goal task quality while using the specified characteristics).

solution. When tackling this problem, 'metaheuristic algorithms' can be classified into four main categories based on their behaviors: 'evolutionary-based', 'physics-based', 'swarm intelligence-based' and 'human-based'. Figure 8.3 depicts the categorization of metaheuristic algorithms.

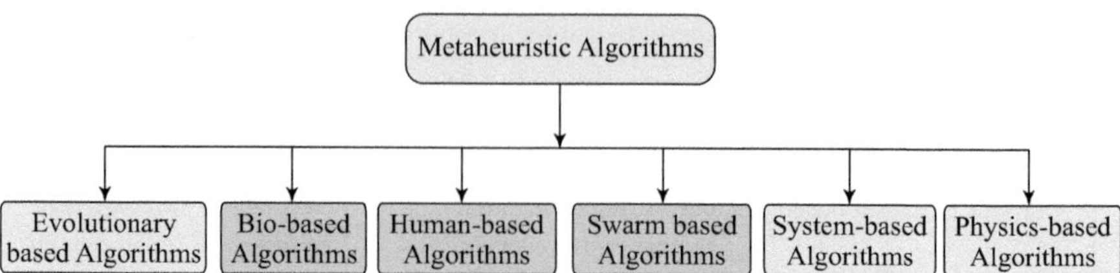

Fig. 8.3   Classification of metaheuristic algorithms

Evolutionary algorithms

It has been noted that there is a lack of focus on this group of algorithms when it comes to addressing the selection of multiclass feature challenges. The finite quantity among such algorithms was currently created, namely between the years 2000 and 2022. The widely used genetics algorithm was integrated using a support vector machine (SVM) classifier to address feature selection challenges and the hospital parameter optimization expenditure model (Tao et al., 2019). This approach applies to both binary and multiclass scenarios. However, the research does not include the specific year it was developed. We have taken this into account in the 'hybrid approach'. Simon presented a 'biogeography-based optimization' technique in 2008 to tackle the real-world issue of choosing sensors to gauge an aircraft engine's health (Simon, 2008). The algorithm's effectiveness was assessed using fourteen standard benchmarks and contrasted with seven based on population optimization methods, such as 'GA', 'DE', 'ACO', 'SGA', and 'PSO'. According to the outcome, BBO and SGA had a superior performance compared to seven out of fourteen standards. The advantages of evolutionary algorithms excel at discovering global optima in intricate search spaces, rendering them ideal for tackling optimization problems that defy traditional methods. They also excel at tackling chaotic or changing environments and effectively handling uncertainties during optimization. This makes them a reliable and robust method for solving complex problems. One disadvantage of evolutionary algorithms is that they may exhibit a slower convergence rate when attempting to find an optimal solution, particularly for intricate problems that involve extensive search spaces. Tuning the parameters of evolutionary algorithms can be a challenging and time-consuming task.

Swarm intelligence

Researchers have directed their attention to swarm-based metaheuristic algorithms progressively. Swarm intelligence systems comprise a collective of simple agents interacting with each other and their local environment. Biological systems, which are commonly observed, tend to derive inspiration from the intricacies of the natural world. The clear benefit in this situation is the 'autonomy' component since the agents function autonomously without external oversight, and every individual agent provides a unique solution to this problem. Moreover, because of this capacity to collaborate, we confidently state that the resilience of this swarm is apparent since it does not possess any one point of weakness.

Another advantage derived from the conduct is 'self-organization'. Prominent methods in the area include 'ant colony optimization' (ACO), 'artificial bee colony' (ABC), 'particle swarm optimization' (PSO) optimization, and others. Various studies have shown that some of these strategies provide satisfactory outcomes in diverse practical scenarios (Kennedy & Eberhart, n.d.). This part describes a comprehensive overview of swarm intelligence metaheuristic algorithms for selecting multiclass classification tasks, including their specific adaptations and the dataset utilized. Although there may be further elements to consider; this clearly illustrates the substantial emphasis on SI during the last two decades. With flexible control architecture, the systems can be easily scaled to accommodate a few or many agents. The systems are highly adaptable, allowing for seamless addition or removal of agents without impacting the overall structure. The systems have a remarkable ability to adapt to new situations quickly. Due to the lack of central control and high redundancy, swarm systems often suffer from inefficiency. Efficient resource allocation is crucial; unfortunately, duplication of effort is a persistent issue. Exerting control over a swarm can be quite challenging. The intricacy of a swarm system can yield unpredictable outcomes.

Ant lion optimizer

'Ant Lion Optimizer' (ALO) simulates the predatory behavior of ant lions in the wild. Mirjalili worked on the creation of this approach in 2015. It includes the development of five critical processes that mirror the hunting behavior of ants. The random movement of the ants, the creation of traps, the capture of prey, the trapping of other ants, and the subsequent rebuilding of the traps are all part of the process (Mirjalili. 2015). M. Wang and fellows proposed a unique strategy in 2019 for feature selection that combines a modified version of ALO called MALO with Weighted Support Vector Machines (WSVM) to successfully decrease the dimensionality of hyperspectral images (M.Wang et al., 2019). Several hyperspectral image datasets were used to compare the MALO method against other existing algorithms. The data revealed that the MALO algorithm performed better than other alternatives (Zawbaa et al., 2016). It provides an effective strategy to overcome feature selection difficulties in their analysis. The investigation focuses on the 'chaotic' variation of the ant-lion optimizer approach. This strategy sought to improve the balance between utilization and investigation stages. For feature selection, the technique passed analysis using several applications of chaotic visualizations to datasets. Medjahed and other authors described techniques in 2023 for choosing essential characteristics and a complete cancer diagnostics methodology using kernel-based learning. To prefilter the genes, the 'SVM recursive feature elimination' (SVM-RFE) method applies. Furthermore, binary dragonfly (BDF) was included in the SVM-RFE. Six microarray datasets from the literature were used in the research. Moreover, the results demonstrated the technique's usefulness, yielding a high accuracy rate of categorization with a smaller collection of genes (Medjahed et al.,

2023). Azar and others have presented a creative search method for the least amount of attribute reduction using ALO and rough sets (Azar et al., 2020). Datasets from the University of California, Irvine (UCI) repository were utilized in the experiment. The experimental results showed that the features selected by ALO were correctly recognized with a fair degree of exactness. This method modified the ALO algorithm and combined it with Le'vy flights to develop the Le'vy Ant-lion Optimization (LALO). This approach was used to pick features in a wrapper-based model. The model aimed to find the best combination of characteristics to improve classification accuracy while decreasing the number of features used. It offers numerous benefits: simplicity, scalability, flexibility, and a well-balanced approach to exploration and exploitation. There are several drawbacks to consider: extended execution time, the tendency to get stuck in local optima, and the risk of premature convergence.

Artificial bee colony algorithm

ABC, or Artificial Bee Colony Algorithm, was designed in 2005 by Dervis Karaboga to improve feature selection in bee colonies. The algorithm combines local and random searches, creating a blended AC-ABC method. The Ant Colony and ABC algorithms were merged to eliminate the ant's immobile behavior and the duration of the worldwide search for novel solutions. The ACO used ABC's utilization skills to choose the top and most significant feature subset, while the bees used the feature subsets produced as a food source (Arya 2022a, 2022b; Arya et al., 2023; A.K. Arya et al., 2022; A.K. Arya, Jain, & Bisht, 2022; A.K. Arya et al., 2022; A.K. Arya & Honwad, 2016, 2018a, 2018b; Adarsh Kumar Arya, 2021, 2022a, 2022c, 2022b; Adarsh Kumar Arya et al., 2022; Adarsh Kumar Arya, Katiyar, et al., 2023; Adarsh Kumar Arya, Kumar, et al., 2023; Adarsh Kumar Arya & Honwad, 2016, 2018a, 2018b; Gupta et al., 2019; Sarkar & Arya, 2022; A.K. Thakur et al., 2021a, 2021b, 2020; Ajit Kumar Thakur et al., 2020, 2022). Thirteen benchmark datasets from the United States Institute of Technology (UCI) were used to test their strategy. A novel 'multi-objective ABC' approach using a feature selection technique was merged with the 'non-dominated' method and 'genetic operators' (Hancer et al., 2018). The binary model method outperformed the constant model by lowering dimensions and obtaining high classification accuracy.

A study by (Zhang and others in 2019) examined the effectiveness of a 'two-archive multi-objective artificial bee colony algorithm' (TMABC-FS), which developed two new algorithms: a diversity-guided search for observer bees and a convergence-guided search for employed bees. The hybrid technique was tested on multiple UCI datasets and compared with conventional algorithms and multi-objective methods (Zhang et al., 2019). Arslan and Ozturk presented a novel strategy in 2019 for choosing features based on ABC Programming (ABCP). Multi Hive ABCP (MHABCP) was used to solve a complex issue with several aspects (Arslan and Ozturk, 2019). FMABC-FS, a quick multi-objective ABC technique, was introduced for feature selection in multiple objectives using evolutionary algorithms (X. Wang et al., 2020). In 2022 Almarzouki used the ABC algorithm to identify a more compact set of genes to classify cancer disorders using Convolutional Neural

Networks (CNNs Almarzouski. 2022). The research provided recommendations on preprocessing and altering gene expression in future studies to augment cancer detection accuracy. It has numerous benefits: Simplicity, flexibility, robustness, the ability to investigate local solutions, and the ability to manage objective costs; implementing this is straightforward and preferred, with its wide range of applications and intricate capabilities. There are several drawbacks: Lack of diversity in the population, a strong focus on searching for equations, and a limited ability to develop new ones.

Bat algorithm

The bat algorithm, inspired by the echolocation activity of bats (Yang and Hossein Gandomi. 2012), has been developed since 2011 and has evolved to address feature selection challenges. The 'binary bat algorithm' (BBA) was introduced by (Nakamura et al., 2012), focusing on binary classification. BANB, a cross between a naive Bayes classifier and a bat algorithm inspired by nature, was suggested and examined using twelve different field datasets (Taha et al., 2013). It outperformed other approaches in picking fewer features while maintaining the precision of categorization and providing further feature subsets. A 'modified bat algorithm' (MBA) was introduced in 2018 to enhance radiofrequency classification for breast cancer diagnosis. The MBA used essential random sampling to select unplanned occurrences and eliminate extraneous characteristics from an initial feature set. However, essential random sampling could be unacceptable in some situations and may lead to information loss.

A 'hybrid BA' version with an enhanced PSO was suggested to strengthen feature selection effectiveness (Tawhid and Dsouza. 2018). The hybridized method's capacity for merging was improved using the PSO algorithm. A KNN classifier-modified 'niche-based bat algorithm' (NBBA) was created to address feature subset selection problems (Saleem et al., 2019). The 'BA' was employed to improve cancer classification accuracy by optimizing feature subset exploration (Hammouri et al., 2020). Wrapper and filter techniques were used to enhance feature selection efficiency. Robust mRMR was employed as a filter approach to identify the most appropriate feature, and the last item wrapping technique used the enhanced BA as its search strategy. There are numerous benefits to this approach. It utilizes straightforward concepts and structure, excels at exploiting opportunities, preserves solution diversity within the population, and boasts of a rapid convergence rate thanks to its ability to focus on promising solutions automatically. The bat algorithm has a common issue of early bat convergence during optimization. This makes it quite challenging to achieve improved optimization results.

Current Issues and Future Trends

- Further investigation is recommended to fully explore the possibilities of the recently suggested approaches, particularly regarding scalability. This is important because in real-world problems, attributes of features and instances tend to grow, and it is crucial to understand how these approaches can handle such growth.

- Reducing computational costs is a critical challenge in the multi-objective feature selection process. It is essential to develop an efficient measure to address this issue. To accomplish this, one must consider two main factors: (1) An efficient search method and (2) Quick evaluation tool.
- A limited number of researchers have investigated the possibility of using dynamic multi-objective techniques to tackle the feature selection problem. For feature selection, it is proposed that the application of dynamic multi-objective optimization may be utilized.
- Suggesting new methods for assessment that could make the fitness landscape less difficult will significantly reduce the issue's challenges and help develop a suitable search technique.

Conclusion

'Multi-objective optimization' using 'recommender systems' is a novel subject that seeks to assist companies and academics in making better choices by maximizing many goals simultaneously. The field blends optimization algorithm abilities with RSs to provide solutions that fulfill competing goals. Multi-Objective Recommender System can influence decision-making in various industries, including e-commerce, healthcare, and transportation. The primary objective of this review is to provide a comprehensive analysis of the current state of research in the field of 'Multi-Objective Reinforcement Learning' (Multi-Objective Recommender System). This review study looks at the various treatments for MORS and offers an overview of the problems and future research prospects.

To accomplish our goal, we conducted a systematic research review that included 'multi-objective optimization' using a recommender system and well-known databases and search phrases. Furthermore, we highlighted the many application domains, techniques employed, apps targeted, performance indicators, and datasets used. Trends were discovered in movies, commodities, travel, web/e-commerce, education, location, code review, applications, and other areas. Evaluation criteria such as diversity, precision, accuracy, recall, 'root means squared error' (RMSE), F1-measure, 'normalized discounted cumulative gain' (NDCG), 'mean average precision' (MAP), coverage, novelty, serendipity, time, fairness, utility, efficiency, distance, and others were also used. Furthermore, we discovered that the datasets utilized in these studies were broad, with popular datasets such as Movie Lens, Book-crossing, Netflix, Speed-Dating, Donation, Google Local, TripAdvisor, and academic datasets being used.

Furthermore, this systematic review study contributes significantly to Multi-Objective Recommender System research. It thoroughly examines existing Multi-Objective Recommender System research, evaluates the merits and limitations of current approaches, and proposes opportunities for future study. We also suggest future research projects that help practitioners who intend employing MORS approaches in real-world applications. Overall, this study will assist researchers, especially novices, in understanding the current limitations and gaps in the area and encourage them to do more research.

References

Almarzouki H.Z. 2022. Deep-Learning-Based Cancer Profiles Classification Using Gene Expression Data Profile. *Journal of Healthcare Engineering*, 2022, 4715998. https://doi.org/10.1155/2022/4715998

Almazini H. and Ku-Mahamud K. 2021. Grey Wolf Optimization Parameter Control for Feature Selection in Anomaly Detection. *International Journal of Intelligent Engineering and Systems*, *14*(2), 474–483. https://doi.org/10.22266/ijies2021.0430.43

Alsaleh A. and Binsaeedan W. 2021. The Influence of Salp Swarm Algorithm-Based Feature Selection on Network Anomaly Intrusion Detection. *IEEE Access, 9*, 112466–112477. https://doi.org/10.1109/access.2021.3102095

Arora S. and Anand P. 2019. Binary butterfly optimization approaches for feature selection. *Expert Systems with Applications, 116*, 147–60. https://doi.org/10.1016/j.eswa.2018.08.051

Arslan S. and Ozturk C. 2019. Multi Hive Artificial Bee Colony Programming for high dimensional symbolic regression with feature selection. *Applied Soft Computing, 78*, 515–27. https://doi.org/10.1016/j.asoc.2019.03.014

Arya A.K. 2022a. A comparison of the MOGA and NSGA-II optimization techniques to reduce the cost of a biomass supply network. *Materials Today: Proceedings.* https://doi.org/10.1016/j.matpr.2021.12.161

Arya A.K. 2022b. A critical review on optimization parameters and techniques for gas pipeline operation profitability. *Journal of Petroleum Exploration and Production Technology, 12*(11). https://doi.org/10.1007/s13202-022-01490-5

Arya A.K., Gautam S. and Yadav S. 2022. Impact of Hydrogen Embrittlement in Pipeline Structures—A Critical Review. In *Springer Proceedings in Materials* (Vol. 15). https://doi.org/10.1007/978-981-19-2572-6_31

Arya A.K. and Honwad S. 2016. Modeling, simulation, and optimization of a high-pressure cross-country natural gas pipeline: Application of an ant colony optimization technique. *Journal of Pipeline Systems Engineering and Practice, 7*(1). https://doi.org/10.1061/(ASCE)PS.1949-1204.0000206

Arya A.K. and Honwad S. 2018a. Multi-objective optimization of a gas pipeline network: an ant colony approach. *Journal of Petroleum Exploration and Production Technology, 8*(4). https://doi.org/10.1007/s13202-017-0410-7

Arya A.K. and Honwad S. 2018b. Optimal Operation of a Multi Source Multi Delivery Natural Gas Transmission Pipeline Network. *Chemical Product and Process Modeling, 13*(3). https://doi.org/10.1515/cppm-2017-0046

Arya A.K., Jain R. and Bisht S. 2022. Corrosion Inhibitors in Oil and Gas Industry—A Critical Review. In *Springer Proceedings in Materials* (Vol. 15). https://doi.org/10.1007/978-981-19-2572-6_27

Arya, A.K. Jain, R., Yadav, S., Bisht, S. and Gautam, S. 2022. Recent trends in gas pipeline optimization. *Materials Today: Proceedings, 57.* https://doi.org/10.1016/j.matpr.2021.11.232

Arya A.K., Katiyar R., Senthil Kumar P., Kapoor A., Pal D.B. et al., 2023. A multi-objective model for optimizing hydrogen injected-high pressure natural gas pipeline networks. *International Journal of Hydrogen Energy.* https://doi.org/10.1016/j.ijhydene.2023.04.133

Arya A.K. 2021. Optimal operation of a multi-distribution natural gas pipeline grid: an ant colony approach. *Journal of Petroleum Exploration and Production Technology, 11*(10), 3859–3878. https://doi.org/10.1007/s13202-021-01266-3

Arya A.K. 2022a. A critical review on optimization parameters and techniques for gas pipeline operation profitability. In *Journal of Petroleum Exploration and Production Technology.* Springer Science and Business Media Deutschland GmbH. https://doi.org/10.1007/s13202-022-01490-5

Arya A.K. 2022c. Application and Challenges of 'Blockchain Technology' in the Oil and Gas Industry. In *Blockchain Technology* (pp. 181–202). https://doi.org/10.1201/9781003138082-11

Arya A.K., Kumar A., Pujari M. and Pacheco D.A.D.J. 2023. Improving natural gas supply chain profitability: A multi-methods optimization study. *Energy*, 128659. https://doi.org/10.1016/j.energy.2023.128659

Aydoğdu Ö. and Ekinci M. 2020. An Approach for Streaming Data Feature Extraction Based on Discrete Cosine Transform and Particle Swarm Optimization. *Symmetry*, *12*(2), 299. https://doi.org/10.3390/sym12020299

Azar A.T., Banu N. and Koubaa A. 2020. Rough Set Based Ant-Lion Optimizer for Feature Selection. In *2020 6th Conference on Data Science and Machine Learning Applications (CDMA)*. IEEE. https://doi.org/10.1109/cdma47397.2020.00020

Balakrishna S., Ganapathiraju A. and Picone J. n.d. Linear discriminant analysis for signal processing problems. In *Proceedings IEEE Southeastcon'99. Technology on the Brink of 2000 (Cat. No.99CH36300)*. IEEE. https://doi.org/10.1109/secon.1999.766096

Chai Z., Li Y. and Zhu S. 2020. P-MOIA-RS: a multi-objective optimization and decision-making algorithm for recommendation systems. *Journal of Ambient Intelligence and Humanized Computing*, *12*(1), 443–54. https://doi.org/10.1007/s12652-020-01997-x

Chen X., Du Y., Xia L. and Wang J. 2021. Reinforcement Recommendation with User Multi-aspect Preference. In *Proceedings of the Web Conference 2021*. ACM. https://doi.org/10.1145/3442381.3449846

Concha-Carrasco J.A., Vega-Rodríguez M.A. and Pérez C.J. 2023. A multi-objective artificial bee colony approach for profit-aware recommender systems. *Information Sciences*, *625*, 476–88. https://doi.org/10.1016/j.ins.2023.01.050

Das P., Das A.K., Nayak J., Pelusi D. and Ding W. 2021. Incremental classifier in crime prediction using bi-objective Particle Swarm Optimization. *Information Sciences*, *562*, 279–303. https://doi.org/10.1016/j.ins.2021.02.002

El-Kenawy E.S.M., Eid M.M., Saber M. and Ibrahim A. 2020. MbGWO-SFS: Modified Binary Grey Wolf Optimizer Based on Stochastic Fractal Search for Feature Selection. *IEEE Access*, *8*, 107635–107649. https://doi.org/10.1109/access.2020.3001151

Emine B.A.Ş. and Ülker E. 2020. An efficient binary social spider algorithm for feature selection problem. *Expert Systems with Applications*, *146*, 113185. https://doi.org/10.1016/j.eswa.2020.113185

Geng S., He X., Liang G., Niu B., Liu S. et al., 2023. Accuracy-diversity optimization in personalized recommender system via trajectory reinforcement based bacterial colony optimization. *Information Processing & Management*, *60*(2), 103205. https://doi.org/10.1016/j.ipm.2022.103205

Ghosh M., Guha R., Sarkar R. and Abraham A. 2019. A wrapper-filter feature selection technique based on ant colony optimization. *Neural Computing and Applications*, *32*(12), 7839–7857. https://doi.org/10.1007/s00521-019-04171-3

Gu Q., Li Z. and Han J. 2011. Correlated multi-label feature selection. In *Proceedings of the 20th ACM international Conference on Information and knowledge management*. ACM. https://doi.org/10.1145/2063576.2063734

Gupta S.S., Arya A.K. and Vijay P. 2019. Designing a model for optimization of maintenance and inspection efforts against third party damage to cross country pipelines in India. *International Journal of Innovative Technology and Exploring Engineering*, *8*(12). https://doi.org/10.35940/ijitee.L3209.1081219

Guyon I. and Elisseeff A. (n.d.). An Introduction to Feature Extraction. In *Feature Extraction* (pp. 1–25). Springer Berlin Heidelberg. https://doi.org/10.1007/978-3-540-35488-8_1

Hammouri A.I., Mafarja M., Al-Betar M.A., Awadallah M.A. and Abu-Doush I. et al., 2020. An improved Dragonfly Algorithm for feature selection. *Knowledge-Based Systems*, *203*, 106131. https://doi.org/10.1016/j.knosys.2020.106131

Hancer E., Xue B., Zhang M., Karaboga D., Akay B. et al., 2018. Pareto front feature selection based on artificial bee colony optimization. *Information Sciences*, *422*, 462–79. https://doi.org/10.1016/j.ins.2017.09.028

Hans R. and Kaur H. 2021. Hybrid Biogeography-Based Optimization and Genetic Algorithm for Feature Selection in Mammographic Breast Density Classification. *International Journal of Image and Graphics, 22*(03). https://doi.org/10.1142/s0219467821400076

Hussain K., Neggaz N., Zhu W. and Houssein E.H. 2021. An efficient hybrid sine-cosine Harris hawks optimization for low and high-dimensional feature selection. *Expert Systems with Applications, 176*, 114778. https://doi.org/10.1016/j.eswa.2021.114778

Kelidari M. and Hamidzadeh J. 2020. Feature selection by using chaotic cuckoo optimization algorithm with levy flight, opposition-based learning and disruption operator. *Soft Computing, 25*(4), 2911–33. https://doi.org/10.1007/s00500-020-05349-x

Kennedy J. and Eberhart R. (n.d.). Particle swarm optimization. In *Proceedings of ICNN'95 - International Conference on Neural Networks*. IEEE. https://doi.org/10.1109/icnn.1995.488968

Li J., Gao Y., Wang K. and Sun Y. 2021. A dual opposition-based learning for differential evolution with protective mechanism for engineering optimization problems. *Applied Soft Computing, 113*, 107942. https://doi.org/10.1016/j.asoc.2021.107942

Lu H., Liu Y., Cheng S. and Shi Y. 2020. Adaptive online data-driven closed-loop parameter control strategy for swarm intelligence algorithm. *Information Sciences, 536*, 25–52. https://doi.org/10.1016/j.ins.2020.05.016

Mafarja M., Aljarah I., Heidari A.A., Faris H., Fournier-Viger P. et al., 2018. Binary dragonfly optimization for feature selection using time-varying transfer functions. *Knowledge-Based Systems, 161*, 185–204. https://doi.org/10.1016/j.knosys.2018.08.003

Mafarja M.M. and Mirjalili S. 2018. Hybrid binary ant lion optimizer with rough set and approximate entropy reducts for feature selection. *Soft Computing, 23*(15), 6249–65. https://doi.org/10.1007/s00500-018-3282-y

Mansour N.A., Saleh A.I., Badawy M. and Ali H.A. 2022. Accurate detection of Covid-19 patients based on Feature Correlated Naïve Bayes (FCNB) classification strategy. *Journal of Ambient Intelligence and Humanized Computing, 13*(1), 41–73. https://doi.org/10.1007/s12652-020-02883-2

Marler R.T. and Arora J.S. 2004. Survey of multi-objective optimization methods for engineering. *Structural and Multidisciplinary Optimization, 26*(6), 369–95. https://doi.org/10.1007/s00158-003-0368-6

Medjahed S.A., Saadi T.A., Benyettou A. and Ouali M. 2023. Corrigendum to "Kernel-based learning and feature selection analysis for cancer diagnosis" [Appl. Soft Comput. 51 (2017) 39–48]. *Applied Soft Computing, 136*, 110098. https://doi.org/10.1016/j.asoc.2023.110098

Mirjalili S. 2015. The Ant Lion Optimizer. *Advances in Engineering Software, 83*, 80–98. https://doi.org/10.1016/j.advengsoft.2015.01.010

Montemayor J.J.M. and Crisostomo R.V. 2019. Feature Selection in Classification using Binary Max-Min Ant System with Differential Evolution. In *2019 IEEE Congress on Evolutionary Computation (CEC)*. IEEE. https://doi.org/10.1109/cec.2019.8790062

Nakamura R.Y.M., Pereira L.A.M., Costa K.A., Rodrigues D., Papa J.P. et al., 2012. BBA: A Binary Bat Algorithm for Feature Selection. In *2012 25th SIBGRAPI Conference on Graphics, Patterns and Images*. IEEE. https://doi.org/10.1109/sibgrapi.2012.47

Peng H., Ying C., Tan S., Hu B. and Sun Z. et al., 2018. An Improved Feature Selection Algorithm Based on Ant Colony Optimization. *IEEE Access, 6*, 69203–69209. https://doi.org/10.1109/access.2018.2879583

Rao H., Shi X., Rodrigue A.K., Feng J., Xia, Y. et al., 2019. Feature selection based on artificial bee colony and gradient boosting decision tree. *Applied Soft Computing, 74*, 634–42. https://doi.org/10.1016/j.asoc.2018.10.036

Rathasamuth W. and Pasupa K. 2019. A Modified Binary Flower Pollination Algorithm: A Fast and Effective Combination of Feature Selection Techniques for SNP Classification. In *2019 11th International Conference on Information Technology and Electrical Engineering (ICITEE)*. IEEE. https://doi.org/10.1109/iciteed.2019.8929963

Renuka Devi D. and Sasikala S. 2019. Online Feature Selection (OFS) with Accelerated Bat Algorithm (ABA) and Ensemble Incremental Deep Multiple Layer Perceptron (EIDMLP) for big data streams. *Journal of Big Data, 6*(1). https://doi.org/10.1186/s40537-019-0267-3

Saleem N., Zafar K. and Sabzwari A. 2019. Enhanced Feature Subset Selection Using Niche Based Bat Algorithm. *Computation, 7*(3), 49. https://doi.org/10.3390/computation7030049

Sarkar A. and Arya A.K. 2022. A Survey on Optimization Parameters and Techniques for Crude Oil Pipeline Transportation. In *Smart Innovation, Systems and Technologies* (Vol. 292). https://doi.org/10.1007/978-981-19-0836-1_43

Sayed G.I., Tharwat A. and Hassanien A.E. 2018. Chaotic dragonfly algorithm: an improved metaheuristic algorithm for feature selection. *Applied Intelligence, 49*(1), 188–205. https://doi.org/10.1007/s10489-018-1261-8

Seymen S., Abdollahpouri H. and Malthouse E.C. 2021. A Constrained Optimization Approach for Calibrated Recommendations. In *Fifteenth ACM Conference on Recommender Systems.* ACM. https://doi.org/10.1145/3460231.3478857

Sharma S. and Kumar V. 2022. A Comprehensive Review on Multi-objective Optimization Techniques: Past, Present and Future. *Archives of Computational Methods in Engineering, 29*(7), 5605–33. https://doi.org/10.1007/s11831-022-09778-9

Simon D. 2008. Biogeography-Based Optimization. *IEEE Transactions on Evolutionary Computation, 12*(6), 702–13. https://doi.org/10.1109/tevc.2008.919004

Sofiane M.A.Z.A. and Zouache D. 2019. Binary Firefly Algorithm for Feature Selection in Classification. In *2019 International Conference on Theoretical and Applicative Aspects of Computer Science (ICTAACS).* IEEE. https://doi.org/10.1109/ictaacs48474.2019.8988137

Taha A.M., Mustapha A. and Chen S.D. 2013. Naive Bayes-guided bat algorithm for feature selection. *The Scientific World Journal, 2013*, 325973. https://doi.org/10.1155/2013/325973

Tan P., Wang X. and Wang Y. 2020. Dimensionality reduction in evolutionary algorithms-based feature selection for motor imagery brain-computer interface. *Swarm and Evolutionary Computation, 52*, 100597. https://doi.org/10.1016/j.swevo.2019.100597

Tao Z., Huiling L., Wenwen W. and Xia Y. 2019. GA-SVM based feature selection and parameter optimization in hospitalization expense modeling. *Applied Soft Computing, 75*, 323–32. https://doi.org/10.1016/j.asoc.2018.11.001

Tawhid M.A. and Dsouza K.B. 2018. Hybrid binary bat enhanced particle swarm optimization algorithm for solving feature selection problems. *Applied Computing and Informatics, 16*(1/2), 117–136. https://doi.org/10.1016/j.aci.2018.04.001

Thakur A.K., Arya A.K. and Sharma P. 2020. The science of alternating current-induced corrosion: a review of literature on pipeline corrosion induced due to high-voltage alternating current transmission pipelines. *Corrosion Reviews, 38*(6). https://doi.org/10.1515/corrrev-2020-0044

Thakur A.K., Arya A.K. and Sharma P. 2021a. Analysis of cathodically protected steel pipeline corrosion under the influence of alternating current. *Materials Today: Proceedings, 50.* https://doi.org/10.1016/j.matpr.2021.05.548

Thakur A.K., Arya A.K. and Sharma P. 2021b. Corrosion of pipe steels under alternating currents. *International Journal of Electrochemical Science, 16.* https://doi.org/10.20964/2021.12.22

Thakur Ajit Kumar, Arya A.K. and Sharma P. 2020. The science of alternating current-induced corrosion: a review of literature on pipeline corrosion induced due to high-voltage alternating current transmission pipelines. *Corrosion Reviews, 38*(6), 463–72. https://doi.org/10.1515/corrrev-2020-0044

Thakur Ajit Kumar, Arya A.K. and Sharma P. 2022. Prediction and mitigation of AC interference on the pipeline system. *Corrosion Reviews.* https://doi.org/10.1515/corrrev-2021-0061

Tran D.H., Leyman P. and De Causmaecker P. 2022. Adaptive passenger-finding recommendation system for taxi drivers with load balancing problem. *Computers & Industrial Engineering, 169*, 108187. https://doi.org/10.1016/j.cie.2022.108187

von Lücken C., Barán B. and Brizuela C. 2014. A survey on multi-objective evolutionary algorithms for many-objective problems. *Computational Optimization and Applications.* https://doi.org/10.1007/s10589-014-9644-1

Vyas J., Das D. and Chaudhury S. 2022. DriveBFR: Driver Behavior and Fuel-Efficiency-Based Recommendation System. *IEEE Transactions on Computational Social Systems, 9*(5), 1446–55. https://doi.org/10.1109/tcss.2021.3112076

Wang M., Wu C., Wang L., Xiang D. and Huang X. et al., 2019. A feature selection approach for hyperspectral image based on modified ant lion optimizer. *Knowledge-Based Systems, 168*, 39–48. https://doi.org/10.1016/j.knosys.2018.12.031

Wang X., Zhang Y., Sun X., Wang Y. and Du C. et al., 2020. Multi-objective feature selection based on artificial bee colony: An acceleration approach with variable sample size. *Applied Soft Computing, 88*, 106041. https://doi.org/10.1016/j.asoc.2019.106041

Wazery Y.M., Saber E., Houssein E.H., Ali A.A., Amer E. et al., 2021. An Efficient Slime Mould Algorithm Combined With K-Nearest Neighbor for Medical Classification Tasks. *IEEE Access, 9*, 113666–113682. https://doi.org/10.1109/access.2021.3105485

Wold S., Esbensen K. and Geladi P. 1987. Principal component analysis. *Chemometrics and Intelligent Laboratory Systems, 2*(1–3), 37–52. https://doi.org/10.1016/0169-7439(87)80084-9

Xue Yani, Li M. and Liu X. 2022. An effective and efficient evolutionary algorithm for many-objective optimization. *Information Sciences, 617*, 211–33. https://doi.org/10.1016/j.ins.2022.10.077

Xue Yu, Jia W. and Liu A.X. 2019. A Particle Swarm Optimization with Filter-based Population Initialization for Feature Selection. In *2019 IEEE Congress on Evolutionary Computation (CEC)*. IEEE. https://doi.org/10.1109/cec.2019.8790156

Yan C., Ma J., Luo H., Zhang G. and Luo J. et al., 2019. A Novel Feature Selection Method for High-Dimensional Biomedical Data Based on an Improved Binary Clonal Flower Pollination Algorithm. *Human Heredity, 84*(1), 34–46. https://doi.org/10.1159/000501652

Yang X. and Hossein Gandomi A. 2012. Bat algorithm: a novel approach for global engineering optimization. *Engineering Computations, 29*(5), 464–83. https://doi.org/10.1108/02644401211235834

Yıldırım E., Azad P. and Gündüz Öğüdücü Ş. 2021. biDeepFM: A multi-objective deep factorization machine for reciprocal recommendation. *Engineering Science and Technology, an International Journal, 24*(6), 1467–77. https://doi.org/10.1016/j.jestch.2021.03.010

Zakeri A. and Hokmabadi A. 2019. Efficient feature selection method using real-valued grasshopper optimization algorithm. *Expert Systems with Applications, 119*, 61–72. https://doi.org/10.1016/j.eswa.2018.10.021

Zawbaa H.M., Emary E. and Grosan C. 2016. Feature Selection via Chaotic Ant-lion Optimization. *PloS One, 11*(3), e0150652–e0150652. https://doi.org/10.1371/journal.pone.0150652

Zhang Y., Cheng S., Shi Y., Gong D., Zhao X. et al., 2019. Cost-sensitive feature selection using two-archive multi-objective artificial bee colony algorithm. *Expert Systems with Applications, 137*, 46–58. https://doi.org/10.1016/j.eswa.2019.06.044

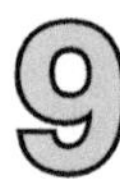

IoT-Blockchain in Remote Pregnancy Care Coordination

Mohammad Mobarak Hossain,[1] Mahruf Islam Prottoy,[2]
Md. Samin Morshed,[3] Dr. Mohammod Abul Kashem,[4]
and Muhammad Usama Islam[5*]

The advent of Remote Pregnancy Monitoring (RPM) stands as a testament to the innovative application of Internet of Things (IoT) and blockchain technologies in the healthcare domain. This paper explores the synergy between IoT devices and blockchain's decentralized architecture to enhance the RPM experience for expectant mothers. We present a systematic review of the current landscape of IoT and blockchain applications in RPM and propose a novel framework that addresses the unique requirements of remote pregnancy care. The proposed RPM framework includes a registration process for expectant mothers and healthcare providers, with their information securely recorded on the blockchain. Smart contracts play a pivotal role in real-time data analysis and in facilitating secure and authenticated access to health data by authorized medical personnel. Our comparative analysis of existing RPM systems focuses on design architectures, data security, data management, consensus methods, and the use of smart contracts. This paper concludes with future research directions, emphasizing the need for scalability, interoperability, and the integration of advanced predictive analytics to further enhance the efficacy of RPM systems for pregnancy care.

[1]   PhD Fellow, DUET, Gazipur, Bangladesh
[2]   Millennium Solutions, Dhaka, Bangladesh
[3]   University of Arkansas at Little Rock, Arkansas, U.S.A.
[4]   Department of Computer Science and Engineering, DUET, Gazipur, Bangladesh
[5]   Asian University of Bangladesh, Bangladesh
*   Corresponding author: usamaislam@iut-dhaka.edu

Introduction

The emergence of blockchain and the Internet of Things (IoT) have had a profound effect on several industries, including healthcare, where they have advanced remote pregnancy care monitoring. The rapid development of wearable IoT medical devices, equipped with diverse functionalities, enables the real-time collection and processing of sensory data from expectant mothers. This data is typically gathered, processed, and kept centrally, which can result in problems including data tampering, single-point failure, and privacy concerns. Because of its decentralized design, blockchain technology can successfully address these problems. Therefore, the amalgamation of IoT and blockchain presents a promising solution for designing a sophisticated remote pregnancy care monitoring system. This study thoroughly examines the body of research that combines blockchain technology with Internet of Things platforms, with a particular emphasis on remote pregnancy care monitoring. We discuss the potential of smart contracts in automating responses and ensuring real-time data analysis within the Remote Patient Monitoring system. Furthermore, we put forth a thorough framework guideline for the Internet of Things based on blockchain technology that tackles design issues, satisfies real-time remote pregnancy care monitoring system needs, and integrates industry best practices discovered in pertinent literature. We outline the future directions for Remote Patient Monitoring systems, emphasizing the need for scalability, interoperability, and advanced analytics to enhance prenatal care. By addressing these key areas, our work aims to contribute to the development of more secure, efficient, and patient-centered Remote Patient Monitoring systems for expectant mothers worldwide.

Improving maternal care could potentially be possible with the growing adoption of Internet of Things (IoT) and blockchain technology in Remote Pregnancy Monitoring (RPM) in healthcare. But currently,there lacks a comprehensive framework that addresses the unique needs of remote pregnancy care in today's environment. In terms of design architectures, data security, data administration, consensus techniques, and the efficient use of smart contracts, this study finds a significant gap in the current RPM systems. These issues must be resolved immediately in order to improve the overall effectiveness and security of RPM systems.

The purpose of this study is to explore and suggest a new framework that best utilizes the interplay between IoT devices and the decentralized nature of blockchain technology. A comprehensive registration procedure for expecting moms and healthcare professionals is part of the planned framework, guaranteeing that their data is safely stored on the blockchain. Smart contracts are recognized as essential elements for enabling safe, authenticated access to health data for authorized medical workers and for real-time data analysis.

A thorough examination of the state of IoT and blockchain applications in RPM will be carried out by this research, with an emphasis on comparative analysis of design architectures, data security protocols, data management strategies, consensus techniques, and the use of smart contracts. By using this data, the study hopes to pinpoint the strengths and weaknesses of the current RPM systems, offering guidance for creating a better framework.

In addition, the study highlights the need to tackle important issues like interoperability and scalability in order to guarantee the smooth integration of sophisticated predictive analytics. The study's conclusion includes a discussion of potential future research avenues, emphasizing the necessity of developments that improve RPM systems' scalability, interoperability, and predictive power in order to further the evolution of safe and efficient remote prenatal care. So, the main contributions of this endeavor is summarized below:

1. Thorough examination of combining blockchain and IoT in remote pregnancy care monitoring.
2. Exploring the potential of smart contracts for automating responses and real-time data analysis.
3. Framework guideline for IoT based on blockchain technology for remote pregnancy care.
4. Integration of industry best practices discovered in pertinent literature.

Thus, our research work is segmented below as the following section provides a comprehensive literature review, followed by several monitoring methods in the next section. How exactly IoT blockchain technology may be complimented is discussed in subsequent sections along with a comprehensive framework and eventually summing up the whole contribution with a final concluding remark.

Literature Review

System Architectures

The utilization of IoT in healthcare has revolutionized patient monitoring by enabling continuous and real-time data collection through wearable devices. These devices, which can be seen as virtual proxies for patients, are equipped with sensors that monitor various health metrics. In the context of remote pregnancy care monitoring, when it comes to monitoring expectant moms' health outside of conventional hospital settings, these technologies are invaluable.

Remote pregnancy care monitoring focuses on expectant mothers who are not hospitalized. It allows healthcare providers to remotely observe and assess the health of these mothers, enabling timely interventions and preventive measures for potential health issues. This form of monitoring relies on the secure collection and storage of health data through IoT devices, which transmit the information to cloud-based systems for healthcare professionals to analyze. In both scenarios, the goal is to provide round-the-clock surveillance to ensure the well-being of patients—or in the case of remote pregnancy care monitoring, the well-being of both the mother and the developing fetus.

A blockchain-based solution was described by (Hasan et al., 2021) and (Griggs et al., 2018), where they utilize smart contracts to provide secure and trustworthy services, as it is a private blockchain system that guarantees the traceability, integrity, and availability of telehealth transactions and data. The former solution features smart contracts for medical diagnostics, medication administration, and teleconsultations; however, the latter solution comes with incorporated consortium and private blockchain networks. Our work in this paper uses a private blockchain for the framework. Tatineni et al., 2020 propose a system that leverages IoT to facilitate better communication and ensures the timely delivery of vaccines and medications, with the goal of reducing mortality rates. This system is akin to our proposed framework, but our work uses more security measures to store and manage patient data using cloud technology, with an emphasis on the privacy and security of sensitive information through the implementation of RSA encryption. Hossain et al., 2023 provide a systematic review of IOT devices in prenatal care which demonstrate potential in improving maternity care by monitoring maternal stress, fetal conditions, and facilitating drug identification and interaction checks.

Treatment for patients benefits substantially from ongoing health monitoring. Because it enables clinicians to monitor patients' conditions from a distance at any time, early detection and prevention of certain illnesses and attacks may be achievable through the system proposed by Archip et al., 2016 and Yew et al., 2016. It should be safe to collect and store patient health data using an Internet of Things-based remote monitoring system. The wearable gadgets read, track, and record various health datasets, which the doctors may then review on the cloud. In the setting of Bangladesh, Ahmed et al., 2021 designed a technique to monitor and forecast pregnant moms' 279 degree of risk in an efficient manner. Using this approach, health data and risk variables for expectant moms will be used to determine the degree of risk intensity. A four-layer system is constructed, according to Jamil et al., 2020, comprising the application layer, IoT blockchain service layer, connectivity layer, and IoT physical layer. Blockchain architecture and services are built at the connectivity layer. They suggested creating a private blockchain network on which only registered and validated entities could communicate, a concept implemented in our work. Pham et al., 2018, suggest an Ethereum-based remote patient monitoring system: patients, physicians, and hospitals. A three-tier design was suggested, with Tier-1—which houses the patient's gateway and IoT devices—using a private blockchain (Badr et al., 2018). At Tier 2, the healthcare providers are connected via a public blockchain. A block of data generated by devices or by patients seeing a provider is added to each person's ledger. Tier-3 hosts the EHR cloud servers, and among them, a public blockchain is used to handle compliance issues. For the management of patient data, a framework was suggested (Abou-Nassar et al., 2020). Based on trusted zones, each member of this model is uniquely identifiable by a signed token. A public blockchain links all peers, where the flaw of this system comes, as public blockchains are inefficient for specialized operations like our paper is working with. A blockchain-based smart contract-based remote patient monitoring system was suggested by Griggs et al., 2018. In its architecture, they have incorporated consortium and private blockchain networks. As a result, in this system, only approved readers can read the block. So, like our work, they have been storing data on cloud storage due to the volume of data.

Security Concerns

In general, IoT Systems face numerous security issues, with various cyber threats posing significant challenges. However, solutions do exist. This section will provide a comprehensive summary of these security issues.

Anita et al., 2019 and Saarikko et al., 2020 showcase the severity of the 51% attack on the systems only, which is not enough to incorporate large scale frameworks like the ones this paper describes. Solat et al., 2017 reveal a solution against selfish mining, called zero block mining, however, this is very specific and does not provide much protection against other attacks. Shakunthala et al., 2018 and De et al., 2016 stress the need of monitoring thresholds in addition to guaranteeing the accuracy of sensor data. A security architecture has been presented by Rathee et al., 2019 for processing multimedia data in healthcare utilizing the blockchain's principle of hashing every piece of data. In their discussion of data accuracy, Cay et al., 2021 suggest sensor validation. Wang et al., 2018 emphasize protection against SQL injection. A scheme of Bayesian Inference-based rating generation is suggested by Yaji et al., 2018 to tackle message spoofing. Ashraf et al., 2018 use Patient-Centric Agent to mitigate DDoS attacks.

Smart Contracts

Smart contracts, when integrated with IoT devices, can significantly enhance remote pregnancy monitoring systems. These self-executing contracts can immediately embed the conditions of the agreement into the code, automating many operations associated with patient monitoring and healthcare delivery. Smart contracts can manage access to sensitive patient data collected by IoT devices. By setting predefined rules, only authorized personnel, such as healthcare providers or the pregnant woman herself, can access the data, ensuring privacy and security. This can be particularly useful in systems like the one proposed by Alotaibi et al., 2018, where patient engagement and information dissemination are key.

How to Monitor Patients

The utilization of IoT in healthcare has fundamentally contributed to a paradigm shift in patient monitoring by enabling continuous and real-time data collection through wearable devices. These devices, which can be seen as virtual proxies for patients, are equipped with sensors that monitor various health metrics. In the context of remote pregnancy care monitoring, these gadgets are essential for monitoring expecting mothers' health outside of conventional hospital settings.

There are two primary environments for patient monitoring: in-hospital and remote. In-hospital monitoring involves patients being monitored within the hospital premises, often with sensors attached to their beds, facilitating constant observation, particularly vital for those in critical care units (Senthamilarasi et al., 2018). This is depicted in Figure 9.1. Remote pregnancy care monitoring, on the other hand, focuses on expectant mothers who are not hospitalized. It allows healthcare

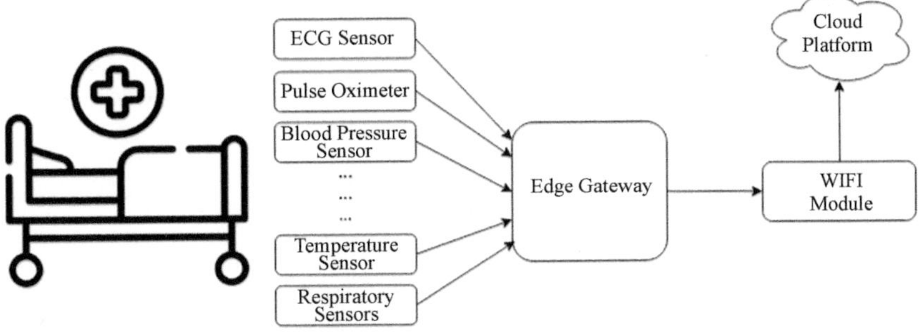

Fig. 9.1   Monitoring in hospital

providers to remotely observe and assess their health enabling timely interventions and preventive measures for potential health issues. This form of monitoring relies on secure collection and storage of health data through IoT devices, which transmit the information to cloud-based systems for healthcare professionals to analyze (Sharma et al., 2017). This is shown in Figure 9.2.

In both scenarios, the goal is to provide round-the-clock surveillance to ensure the well-being of patients—or in the case of remote pregnancy care monitoring, the well-being of both the mother and the developing fetus.

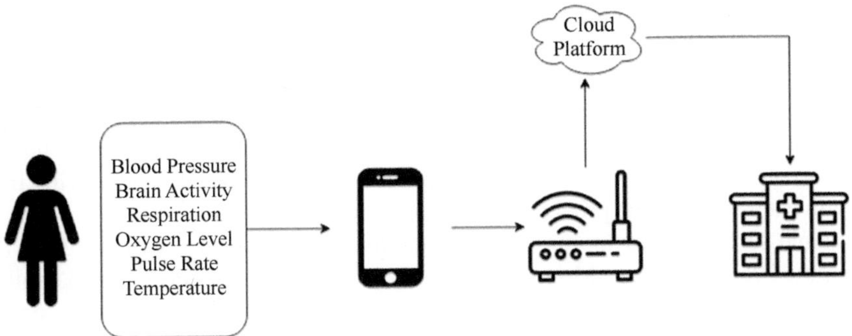

Fig. 9.2   Monitoring remotely

IoT and Blockchain in Remote Pregnancy Care

These systems integrate blockchain technology with IoT to improve the scalability as well as the dependability of IoT systems (Reyna et al., 2018). Blockchain ensures data integrity and anonymity while processing and storing a variety of data types. Autonomous interaction in IoT-based systems is one of the blockchain's smart contract features (Dai et al., 2019). Thus, IoT-Blockchain is an effective and user-friendly solution for Remote Pregnancy Care Monitoring.

Design Challenges

The creation of an IoT system with an eventual blockchain based security integration for remote prenatal care monitoring presents several difficulties for developers to overcome. These critical design challenges include:

Information Delay

Remote Pregnancy Care Monitoring patients are in different geographical areas, resulting in potential network delays in collecting data from their sensors. Managing information delay becomes a major difficulty because the system demands constant data collecting and functions in real-time.

Data Security

Ensuring health data security is of utmost importance, as tampered data could mislead doctors and compromise patient treatment. The Remote Pregnancy Care Monitoring system must incorporate robust authentication techniques to safeguard the collected and stored data.

Scalability

Scalability is a crucial consideration for a Remote Pregnancy Care Monitoring system, especially as it aims to alleviate the workload of healthcare professionals by monitoring numerous patients. As the number of patients within the system increases, ensuring that the system can accommodate this growth without compromising its performance becomes imperative. To achieve scalability, developers must implement measures and strategies that allow the system to handle the expanding network and maintain optimal functionality efficiently. This may involve optimizing data processing, enhancing network infrastructure, and adopting scalable technologies to support the increasing demand and workload on the Remote Pregnancy Care Monitoring system. By effectively addressing scalability challenges, the system can sustainably grow and continue to provide reliable remote patient monitoring services to a larger population of patients.

Storage

The system generates a constant stream of data, necessitating the storage of large volumes of information. Effective data management techniques are needed to deal with the limited storage capacity of IoT devices.

Anonymity of Data

Patient data stored within the system must maintain strict anonymity to protect patient privacy. In the event of a security breach, maintaining data anonymity can reduce potential harm to the patients. Constant Monitoring: Each patient's health condition, medical history, and health issues are unique. The Remote Pregnancy Care Monitoring system must be capable of handling this heterogeneity in real-time and provide alerts for emergencies to both the medical staff and the patient.

Framework for the Remote Pregnancy Care Monitoring System

The IoT Blockchain-based system relies on a blockchain network to establish connections between physicians and patients. Every data exchange occurs within the network. An important feature of distributed ledger technology is that the data entered into the blockchain becomes accessible to all peers in the network. As a result, all participants can access the same information, ensuring transparency and fostering trust in the RPM system. A rundown of the framework is depicted in Figure 9.3.

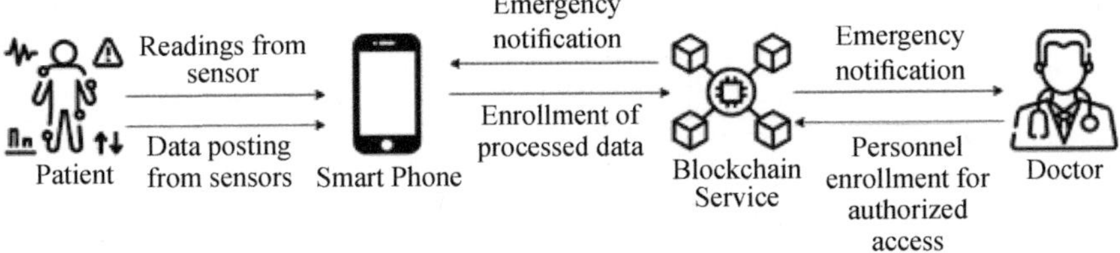

Fig. 9.3   Remote pregnancy care monitoring framework

Patients and doctors are the two user categories that make up the system. Both groups connect to the platform through cell phones. It is structured as a distributed network enhanced by incorporating a blockchain induced network inside the core of the network layer. The distributed ledger technology is fully functional on this blockchain network, which gives the system an additional degree of security and transparency.

Framework Guidelines

We have examined IoT-based blockchain solutions within the Remote Pregnancy care monitoring area in this article. We noted that the focus regions of various solutions vary. For instance, some concentrate on blockchain technology, others on architecture, data security and administration, and more. We have found that there is a deficiency remains in the literature for a thorough framework that unifies disparate elements. We provide a thorough framework of guidelines in this section t. This recommendation was created after we examined the benefits and drawbacks of the current frameworks while considering the difficulties posed by IoT-Blockchain in the monitoring system.

Framework Components

The proposed framework for remote pregnancy monitoring encompasses three distinct user groups: expectant mothers, healthcare providers, and medical facilities.

Within this framework, each expectant mother is considered a node within the network, with various IoT devices attached to her body to monitor health metrics. These devices are crucial for collecting and transmitting health data to the associated medical facility responsible for the mother's prenatal care. The key elements of this framework are outlined as follows:

Expectant Mothers

They are integrated into the network as individual nodes. Wearable IoT devices are placed on them to continuously monitor their health and transmit data to the healthcare system.

Healthcare Providers: Doctors and other medical professionals are users who can access and interpret the health data collected from the IoT devices placed on expectant mothers. They make educated decisions on the moms' health and the necessary prenatal care using this information.

Medical Facilities

Clinics and hospitals are regarded as the primary hubs for organizing and managing patient health data. They are in charge of monitoring expected women's health and making sure that the information gathered is safe and properly utilized for tracking and treatment.

Blockchain Integration

A blockchain induced network is incorporated that connects each component of the system's elements. Verifying each node's addition to the network is essential. Since the data must be accessible to all users, the network operates on a permissioned peer-to-peer blockchain. There are no nodes roaming throughout the network thanks to the blockchain. Because there are no malicious nodes in the system, the PBFT consensus mechanism should ensure the validity of each transaction in the network. Instead of being directly stored on the blockchain, healthcare data is obtained and saved through transactions. A cloud server is where the processed patient data ought to be kept. To provide safe data access, all users should have access to digital signatures. Each transaction must be connected to many smart contracts to follow it in real time. They will activate in response to data values and peer behavior.

Cloud Storage

The volume of healthcare data increases with time due to the continual collection of monitoring data and the requirement for its storage. If the data exists in a blockchain ledger, a huge amount of storage will be needed. Furthermore, data unavailability may arise from a node's disconnection if we need to keep the pertinent data inside the blockchain. So, as part of the transaction, the real data can be stored on cloud. The network will eventually store it through a link.

Operations

This section for Remote Pregnancy Care Monitoring outlines the critical procedures within the system, focusing on three principal operations (Figure 9.4):

Registration

Physicians and expected mothers will submit registration requests and provide the hospital with all the necessary information (Task 1.1, Figure 9.4). Afterwards, via a specific smart contract in the system, the hospital authorities will verify them. (Task 1.2, Figure 9.4). Patient and physician data will be added to the blockchain's ledger upon validation by the smart contracts (Task 1.3, Figure 9.4). Finally, a patient will be paired with a doctor by the hospital administration (Task 1.4, Figure 9.4).

Data Storage while Monitoring

Each health data point is constantly gathered, recorded, and kept in the system; any anomalous occurrence must be reported to the relevant parties. The patient's smartphone or tablet will receive raw sensor and device readings through a mobile application (Task 2.1, Figure 9.4). After that, the unprocessed data will be formatted and handled by the mobile application (Task 2.2, Figure 9.4). Following processing, a specific smart contract is applied to the data for further analysis (Task 2.3, Figure 9.4). Based on monitoring data, we can develop smart contracts so that it allows them to recognize any abnormal patient states since the system needs to be monitored in real-time. These should stay on the cloud storage platform after the data from the smart contract is examined (Task 2.4, Figure 9.4). Each event involving the upload or access of data must be documented as a transaction in the ledger. It is recommended that cloud storage be used to store all data from the patient being monitored. and comply with HIPAA requirements to guarantee that there is no way to link the data to any patient (Task 2.5, Figure 9.4). To take immediate action if the smart contract detects an abnormal state during analysis, the patient, doctor, and hospital must all be notified (Task 2.6, Figure 9.4).

Data Retrieval

Another essential feature of the system is its ability for doctors to view or retrieve monitoring data particular to a given patient. The patient must give the doctor their key in order to request access to their data. (Task 3.1, Figure 9.4). Upon receiving a request into the system from the doctor, before the doctor's validity is established, a smart contract will be initiated to grant permission to the patient's data (Task 3.2, Figure 9.4). Once the patient has been verified in the system, the relevant stakeholder, which in this case is a doctor, can acquire from the ledger the pertinent health data provided by the patient (Task 3.3, Figure 9.4).

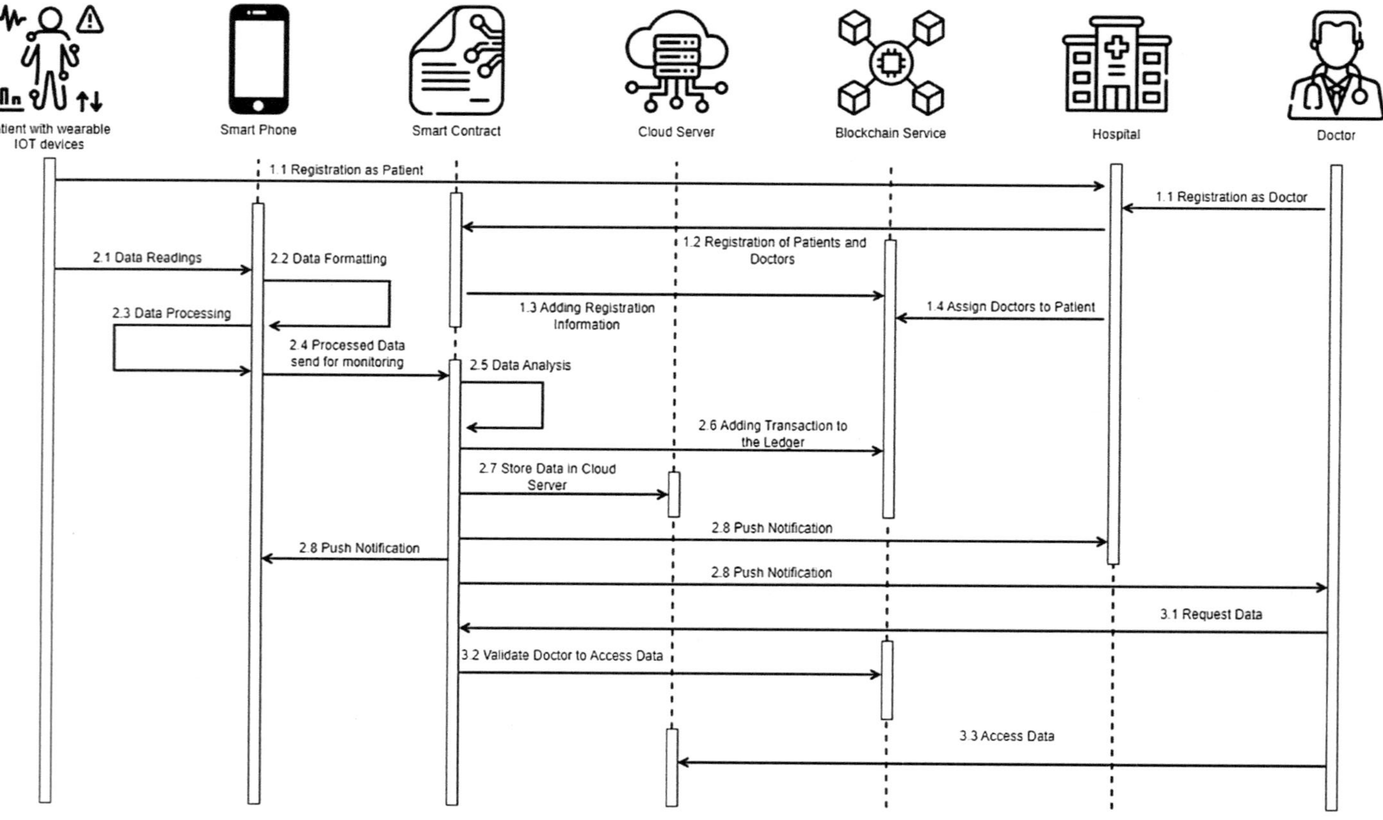

Fig. 9.4   Operations of the framework

Limitations

The research faces several notable limitations, including "information delay in collecting data from sensors," which could introduce temporal gaps and compromise the timeliness of data acquisition. Additionally, concerns arise regarding "data security and authentication techniques," as vulnerabilities in these areas may pose risks to the confidentiality and integrity of the collected information. Another constraint is the "scalability to handle increasing numbers of patients," raising questions about the system's ability to efficiently manage a growing volume of data. "Maintaining strict anonymity of patient data" emerges as a critical concern, as any lapses in anonymity protection could have ethical and legal ramifications. Lastly, the challenge of implementing "real-time monitoring and alerts for emergencies" adds complexity, potentially impacting the system's responsiveness in critical situations. Addressing these limitations is imperative to enhance the overall robustness and reliability of the research outcomes.

Conclusion

To sum up, the combination of blockchain technology and IOT presents a splendid chance to enhance Remote Pregnancy Care Monitoring systems. As covered in this paper, the suggested methodology provides a strong framework for effectively and safely handling expecting mothers' health data. The solution guarantees that healthcare practitioners may give prompt and customized care to their patients by utilizing the decentralized nature of blockchain technology and the real-time data collection capabilities of IoT devices.

Going forward, future work should concentrate on improving these technologies' scalability and compatibility. The system needs to have the ability to accommodate expansion in both user count and data volume without sacrificing security or performance. Furthermore, for broad adoption, user-friendly interfaces and smooth integration with the current healthcare infrastructure would be essential. It will also be crucial to ensure adherence to international data privacy laws and to resolve any ethical issues pertaining to patient data. Pilot studies and clinical trials will be crucial as the technology develops to confirm the system's efficacy and adjust its constituent parts for best results.

In essence, the continuous evolution of Remote Pregnancy Care Monitoring systems revolutionize prenatal care, ensuring accessible, efficient, and effective care for expectant mothers around the world. Essentially, the ongoing development of remote pregnancy care monitoring systems has the potential to completely transform prenatal care, increasing its effectiveness, efficiency, and accessibility for pregnant moms at any location.

References

Abou-Nassar E.M., Iliyasu A.M., Elkafrawy P., Song O., Bashir A.K. et al., 2020. DITRUST Chain: Towards blockchain-based trust models for sustainable healthcare IoT systems. *IEEE Access*, 8, 111223–111238. https://doi.org/10.1109/access.2020.2999468

Ahmed M. and Kashem M.A. 2020. IoT based risk level prediction model for maternal health care in the context of Bangladesh. In 2020 2nd International Conference on Sustainable Technologies for Industry 4.0 (STI), 1-6. IEEE. https://doi.org/10.1109/sti50764.2020.9350320

Alotaibi M., Albalawi M. and Alwakeel L. 2018. A smart mobile pregnancy management and awareness system for Saudi Arabia. *International Journal of Interactive Mobile Technologies*, 12(5), 112. https://doi.org/10.3991/ijim.v12i5.9005

Anita N. and Vijayalakshmi M. 2019. Blockchain security attack: A brief survey. In 2019 10th International Conference on Computing, Communication and Networking Technologies (ICCCNT), Kanpur, India, 2019, 1-6. IEEE. https://doi.org/10.1109/icccnt45670.2019.8944615

Archip A., Botezatu N., Şerban E., Herghelegiu P. and Zala A. 2016. An IoT-based system for remote patient monitoring. 2016 17th International Carpathian Control Conference (ICCC), 2016, 1–6. https://doi.org/10.1109/carpathiancc.2016.7501056

Badr S., Gomaa I.A. and Abd-Elrahman E. 2018. Multi-tier blockchain framework for IoT-EHRs systems. *Procedia Computer Science*, 141, 159–166. https://doi.org/10.1016/j.procs.2018.10.162

Cay G., Solanki D., Ravichandran V., Hoffman L., Laptook A.R. et al., 2021. Baby-guard: An IoT-based neonatal monitoring system integrated with smart textiles. In 2021 IEEE International Conference on Smart Computing (SMARTCOMP). IEEE. https://doi.org/10.1109/smartcomp52413.2021.00038

Dai H., Zheng Z. and Zhang Y. 2019. Blockchain for internet of things: A survey. *IEEE Internet of Things Journal*, 6(5), 8076–8094. https://doi.org/10.1109/jiot.2019.2920987

De D., Mukherjee A., Sau A. and Bhakta I. 2016. Design of smart neonatal health monitoring system using SMCC. Healthcare Technology Letters, 4(1), 13–19. https://doi.org/10.1049/htl.2016.0054

Griggs K.N., Ossipova O., Kohlios C.P., Baccarini A.N., Howson E.A. et al., 2018. Healthcare blockchain system using smart contracts for secure automated remote patient monitoring. *Journal of Medical Systems*, 42(7). https://doi.org/10.1007/s10916-018-0982-x

Hasan H.R., Salah K., Jayaraman R., Yaqoob I., Omar M. et al., 2021. Blockchain-enabled telehealth services using smart contracts. *IEEE Access*, 9, 151944–151959. https://doi.org/10.1109/access.2021.3126025

Hossain M.M., Kashem M.A., Islam M.M., Sahidullah M., Mumu S.H. et al., 2023. Internet of things in pregnancy care coordination and management: A systematic review. *Sensors*, 23(23), 9367. https://doi.org/10.3390/s23239367

Jamil F., Ahmad S., Iqbal N. and Kim D. 2020. Towards a remote monitoring of patient vital signs based on IoT-based blockchain integrity management platforms in smart hospitals. *Sensors*, 20(8), 2195. https://doi.org/10.3390/s20082195

Masi S., Banu R.J., Deepika L. and Indu R. 2018. Neonatal healthcare monitoring in incubator using IoT. *International Journal of Electrical, Electronics and Data Communication*, 6(6), 59–64. https://www.researchgate.net/publication/344217643

Pham H.L., Tran T.H. and Nakashima Y. 2018. A secure remote healthcare system for hospital using blockchain smart contract. 2018 IEEE Globecom Workshops, Abu Dhabi, United Arab Emirates, 2018. https://doi.org/10.1109/glocomw.2018.8644164

Rathee G., Sharma A., Saini H., Kumar R. and Iqbal R. et al., 2019. A hybrid framework for multimedia data processing in IoT-healthcare using blockchain technology. Multimedia Tools and Applications, 79(15–16), 9711–33. https://doi.org/10.1007/s11042-019-07835-3

Reyna A., Martin C.L., Chen J., Soler E. and Díaz M. et al., 2018. On blockchain and its integration with IoT: Challenges and opportunities. *Future Generation Computer Systems*, 88, 173–90. https://doi.org/10.1016/j.future.2018.05.046

Saarikko J., Niela-Vilén H., Ekholm E., Hamari L., Azimi I. et al., 2020. Continuous 7-month internet of things–based monitoring of health parameters of pregnant and postpartum women:

Prospective observational feasibility study. *JMIR Formative Research*, 4(7), e12417. https://doi. org/10.2196/12417

Senthamilarasi C., Rani J.J., Vidhya B. and Aritha H. 2018. A smart patient health monitoring system using IoT. *International Journal of Pure and Applied Mathematics*, 119(16), 59–70. http://www. acadpubl.eu/hub/Special Issue

Sharma P.K., Singh S., Jeong Y.S. and Park J.H. 2017. DistBlockNet: a distributed blockchains-based secure SDN architecture for IoT networks. IEEE Communications Magazine, 55(9), 78–85. https:// ieeexplore.ieee.org/abstract/document/8030491

Solat S. and Potop-Butucaru M. 2017. Brief announcement: Zeroblock: Timestamp-free prevention of block-withholding attack in bitcoin. In Lecture Notes in Computer Science (pp. 356–60). https:// doi.org/10.1007/978-3-319-69084-1_25

T, S.B., Bdj A., N M.S., Devi R.S., Thenmozhi V., Amirtharajan R. et al., 2020. IoT with light weight crypto system for primary health centers to minimize fetus death, birth defects and premature delivery in Solamadevi village Trichy district. 2020 International Conference on Computer Communication and Informatics (ICCCI), 1–4. https://doi.org/10.1109/iccci48352.2020.9104180

Uddin M.A., Stranieri A., Gondal I. and Balasubramanian V. 2018. Continuous patient monitoring with a patient centric agent: a block architecture. *IEEE Access*, 6, 32700–32726. https://doi. org/10.1109/access.2018.2846779

Wang S., Zhu S. and Zhang Y. 2018. Blockchain-based mutual authentication security protocol for distributed RFID systems. In 2018 IEEE Symposium on Computers and Communications (ISCC), 2018. IEEE. https://doi.org/10.1109/iscc.2018.8538567

Yaji S., Bangera K. and Neelima B. 2018. Privacy preserving in blockchain based on partial homomorphic encryption system for AI applications. In 2018 IEEE 25th International Conference on High Performance Computing Workshops (HiPCW), Bengaluru, India, 2018. IEEE. https://doi. org/10.1109/hipcw.2018.8634280

Yew H.T., Ng M.F., Ping S.Z., Chung S.K., Chekima A. et al., 2020. IoT based real-time remote patient monitoring system. 2020 16th IEEE International Colloquium on Signal Processing & Its Applications (CSPA), Langkawi, Malaysia, 2020, 176–79. https://doi.org/10.1109/ cspa48992.2020.9068699

10

Strengthening Healthcare Data Security and Privacy

Vibha Jain[1] and *Rohit Singh*[2*]

The potential of blockchain technology to revolutionize a variety of industries, including healthcare, has attracted a lot of interest in recent years. Healthcare data possesses the risk of cyber-attacks and a peer-to-peer decentralized blockchain network can help achieve security, transparency, interoperability, and privacy. The amalgamation of blockchain technology with electronic health records has stirred up the traditional medical record system. In this chapter, we investigate how blockchain technology may be used to create a safe healthcare infrastructure. We have studied different use cases of blockchain in healthcare, including data interoperability, patient identity management, electronic health records, and clinical trials. Additionally, the discussion also includes the difficulties and factors to be considered when deploying blockchain in healthcare, including scalability, legal compliance, system integration, and ethical issues. Future directions and research prospects include new patterns and the incorporation of cutting-edge technology like AI and smart contracts in blockchain-based healthcare. The chapter concludes by highlighting the importance of blockchain in safeguarding healthcare systems and outlining a path for its implementation and its future effects.

Introduction

The healthcare sector encounters a multitude of obstacles in effectively managing and safeguarding patient data, all the while striving to facilitate seamless data

[1]   Thapar Institute of Engineering and Technology Patiala, India.
[2]   Manipal University, Jaipur, India.
*   Corresponding author: rohit.singh@jaipur.manipal.edu

exchange and collaboration among various entities involved. The vulnerability of traditional centralized systems to data breaches has been well-documented, resulting in compromised patient privacy and insufficient data integrity. In recent times, the utilization of blockchain technology has emerged as a promising remedy to tackle these pressing concerns, presenting a decentralized, transparent, and secure framework for the management of healthcare data (Pandey and Litoriya, 2020).

Blockchain technology, which was initially created for digital currencies such as Bitcoin, is a decentralized ledger that documents transactions or data entries across numerous nodes or computers (Shahnaz et al., 2019). The system functions based on the fundamental principles of decentralization, immutability, and cryptographic security. Every individual transaction or data entry, referred to as a block, is sequentially connected to the preceding block, forming a chronological sequence of interconnected blocks. The utilization of this framework guarantees transparency, as all individuals within the network are granted equal access to the identical iteration of the blockchain, thereby obviating the necessity for intermediaries and central governing bodies (Kumar et al., 2022).

The healthcare industry can derive numerous advantages from the decentralized nature of blockchain technology. One significant benefit is the improvement of data security. By distributing data across multiple nodes, blockchain mitigates the risk of a single point of failure and makes it exceedingly difficult for hackers to alter or tamper with the data (Xie et al., 2021). Additionally, blockchain employs cryptographic algorithms to encrypt data, ensuring that only authorized parties can access and decrypt sensitive information. This heightened security measure can safeguard patient records, clinical trial data, and other confidential healthcare information (Chen et al., 2019).

Data integrity is another critical aspect addressed by blockchain technology. The immutability of blockchain ensures that once a transaction is recorded, it cannot be altered or deleted without the consensus of the network participants. This feature is particularly valuable in healthcare, where the integrity of medical records and clinical data is of utmost importance. Interoperability and data exchange are significant challenges within the healthcare ecosystem. The fragmented nature of healthcare systems, with various entities using different electronic health record (EHR) systems, hinders seamless data sharing and collaboration (Pandey and Litoriya, 2020). Blockchain can enable secure and efficient data exchange by establishing a standardized framework for interoperability. It provides a trusted platform where different healthcare organizations can securely share and access patient data while ensuring data privacy and consent.

Moreover, blockchain technology has the potential to empower patients by giving them greater control over their health information. With blockchain-based solutions, individuals can securely store and manage their medical records, granting selective access to healthcare providers, researchers, and other relevant parties. This patient-centric approach fosters data ownership and empowers patients to actively participate in their healthcare decisions (Cheng et al., 2020). With blockchain, healthcare providers can maintain a transparent and auditable trail of data, allowing for better traceability and accountability.

Significance of Blockchain in Healthcare

There are several ways in which blockchain technology might improve the healthcare system.

- Blockchain's distributed ledger architecture makes it more difficult to exploit a single point of failure and improves data integrity.
- Blockchain's immutability preserves data integrity by shielding it from unauthorized changes to the ledger.
- Blockchain has the potential to build a standard framework for the safe and efficient interchange of data across healthcare organizations, which is known as interoperability.
- Blockchain-based solutions provide patients more agency by putting them in charge of their own health records and data.

Current Challenges in Healthcare Security

The healthcare sector today needs to construct a more secure, transparent, and patient-centric data management system and can do so with the help of blockchain technology by addressing the following issues.

- Traditional centralized systems may be breached, putting patients' personal information and medical records at risk (Qiu et al., 2018).
- Problems with interoperability arise when different organizations use different electronic health record (EHR) systems, preventing useful information from being shared and limiting opportunities for cooperation (Fu et al., 2020).
- Constantly changing cyber risks need increased spending on healthcare network security (Qiu et al., 2018).
- Medical records and other health data must be accurate and trustworthy, but this may be difficult to ensure without an auditable and accessible trail (McGhin et al., 2019).
- Patients' lack of authority over their own health information is a major barrier to their full and equal involvement in all aspects of healthcare decision-making (McGhin et al., 2019).

Blockchain Fundamentals and Applications in Health Industry

Fundamentals of Blockchain Technology

Blockchain technology is a distributed ledger that is decentralized and has grown very popular because of its ability to safeguard and verify transactions without the need for a central authority. Although it was first developed to power the cryptocurrency Bitcoin, its uses have now gone much beyond the financial industry.

By guaranteeing openness, immutability, and trust among network participants, blockchain offers a revolutionary method of data management (Adere. 2022). These are the essential elements of a blockchain network as presented in Figure 10.1 and the structure of the blockchain is presented in Figure 10.2.

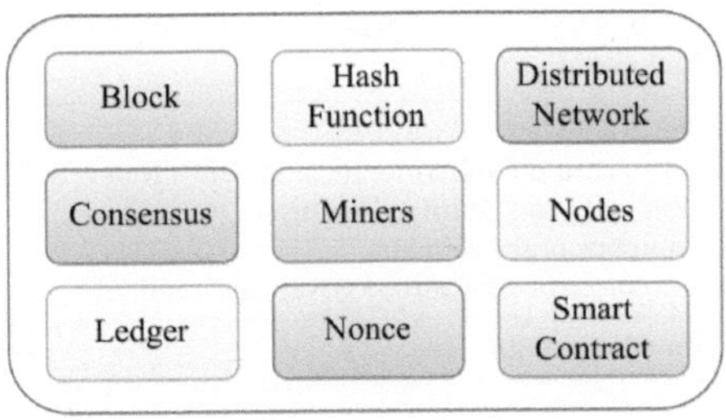

Fig. 10.1   Components of blockchain

- *Blocks:*   A blockchain is made up of a series of blocks, each of which has a certain set of transactions. By employing cryptographic hashing to connect these blocks, an unchangeable record of the data is produced.
- *Hash Function:*   A fixed-length string created from the data in a block is called a cryptographic hash, and it is present in every block. This hash is essential for maintaining the blockchain's integrity.
- *Distributed Network:*   Every node in the decentralized network of nodes used by blockchain to run it keeps a copy of the complete blockchain. With this distribution, redundancy is guaranteed, and the system's resistance to errors or assaults is strengthened.
- *Consensus Protocol:*   Blockchains employ consensus procedures to verify and concur on the contents of each block. Without the aid of a centralized authority, these protocols make a guarantee that all network nodes can agree on the blockchain's current state.

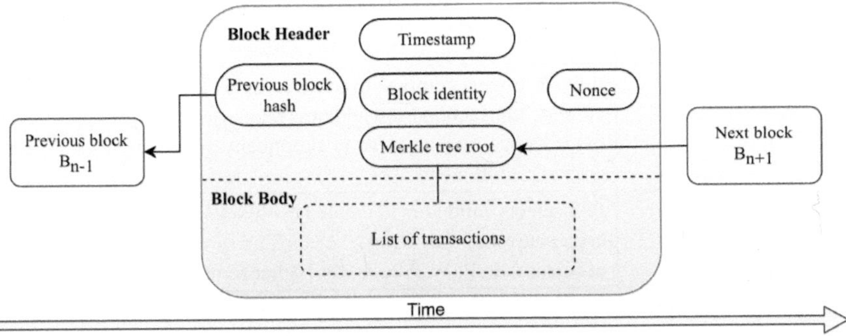

Fig. 10.2   Structure of blockchain

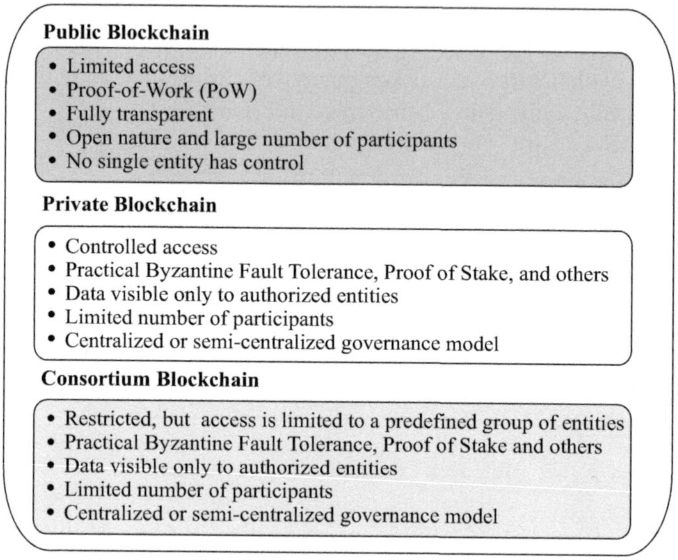

Public Blockchain

- Limited access
- Proof-of-Work (PoW)
- Fully transparent
- Open nature and large number of participants
- No single entity has control

Private Blockchain

- Controlled access
- Practical Byzantine Fault Tolerance, Proof of Stake, and others
- Data visible only to authorized entities
- Limited number of participants
- Centralized or semi-centralized governance model

Consortium Blockchain

- Restricted, but access is limited to a predefined group of entities
- Practical Byzantine Fault Tolerance, Proof of Stake and others
- Data visible only to authorized entities
- Limited number of participants
- Centralized or semi-centralized governance model

Fig. 10.3   Types of blockchain

As shown in Figure 10.3, blockchain technology is categorized into three main groups: Public, private, and consortium blockchains. Each type serves different purposes and has distinct characteristics. Public blockchains are open and permissionless, allowing anyone to participate in and validate transactions (Prybutok et al., 2022). Private blockchains, on the other hand, are permissioned and restrict access to specific individuals or entities, making them more suitable for business use cases that prioritize data privacy. Consortium blockchains combine elements of both public and private blockchains, where a pre-selected group of entities set the consensus rules and access controls (Pradhan et al., 2022). A comprehensive overview of the various consensus mechanisms used in blockchain technology, are as presented in Table 10.1.

Table 10.1   Consensus mechanisms in blockchain technology.

Consensus Mechanism	*Description*
Proof-of-Work (PoW)	In PoW, miners compete to solve complex mathematical puzzles to validate transactions and add new blocks to the blockchain. Secure but resource-intensive due to significant computational power and energy requirements.
Proof-of-Stake (PoS)	PoS selects validators to create new blocks based on the amount of cryptocurrency they "stake" or lock up as collateral. More energy-efficient than PoW. Allows for higher transaction throughput.
Delegated Proof-of-Stake (DPoS)	DPoS is a variation of PoS where token holders vote for delegates who validate transactions and produce new blocks. Aims to increase efficiency by reducing the number of validators.

Table Contd.

Practical Byzantine Fault Tolerance (PBFT)	PBFT is suitable for permissioned blockchains and relies on a predefined group of validators exchanging messages to agree on the order of transactions.
Proof of Concept and Pilots	Conducting POC and pilot projects provides valuable insights and helps identify potential challenges before full-scale deployment.
Continual Evaluation and Improvement	Regular evaluation of performance, security, and user experience ensures the long-term relevance and effectiveness of the solution.

Blockchain Applications in Healthcare

In this section, key applications of blockchain in the domain of healthcare are discussed.

- *Data Interoperability:* The term "data interoperability" is used to describe the safe and efficient transfer of patient data across various parties involved in the healthcare industry when using blockchain technology. Blockchain makes standardized, near-instantaneous data exchange possible because of its decentralized nature, consensus processes, and smart contracts. Patients may manage who has access to their data thanks to security and privacy measures (Saidi et al., 2022). In the healthcare sector, blockchain improves interoperability by eliminating data silos and boosting productivity, precision, and service to patients, Figure 10.4 shows its basic working.

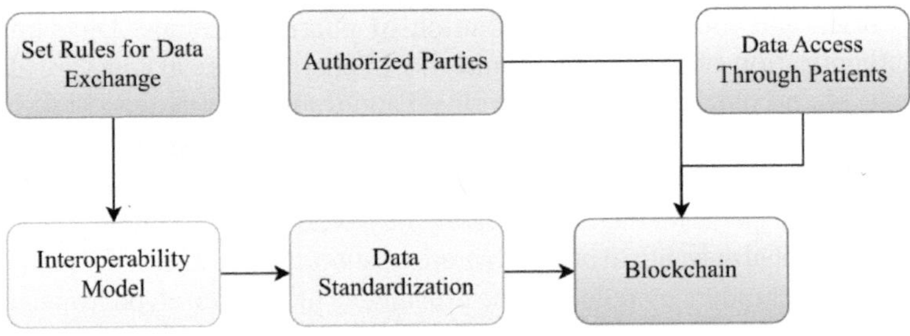

Fig. 10.4   Data interoperability model

- *Identity Management:* Securely and effectively managing patient IDs and access to healthcare services is a key use case for blockchain's identity management functionality in healthcare applications. The immutability and decentralization of the blockchain record keep personal information safe and secure. By assigning each patient a distinct digital identity that is securely recorded on the blockchain and verifiable by authorized healthcare professionals, we can expedite the registration process, cut down on fraud, and enhance the quality of treatment we give. The healthcare ecosystem benefits from increased trust and transparency thanks to blockchain-powered identity management's focus on providing a more secure, interoperable, and patient-centric approach to treatment (Villarreal et al., 2023).

- *Electronic health records (EHRs):*   To better store, manage, and communicate patient medical information, blockchain technology is being used in the realm of Electronic Health Records (EHRs). Due to its distributed and immutable nature, blockchain technology improves data security, integrity, and privacy. While patients retain ownership of their data, authorized healthcare professionals have instant access to their most up-to-date EHRs through the blockchain. Better patient care and results are the goal of blockchain-powered EHRs, which seek to increase data interoperability, decrease medical mistakes, boost patient involvement, and simplify healthcare operations (Lakhan et al., 2023).

- *Clinical trials and research data management:*   Blockchain technology is being investigated for its potential use in handling clinical studies and research data in the context of healthcare applications. The adoption of blockchain has benefits, including better data security, integrity, and accessibility for all parties involved. Data security, privacy, and interoperability are three problems that blockchain-based applications for healthcare want to solve by creating a distributed, immutable ledger. Current research and development indicate excellent promises for revolutionizing study and research data management in the healthcare business, despite constraints like scalability, privacy issues, integration, and regulatory compliance (Gupta et al., 2023).

- *Supply chain and pharmaceutical tracking:*   Supply chain and pharmaceutical tracking in healthcare uses of blockchain include using blockchain technology to track and monitor the distribution of pharmaceuticals. Data integrity, authentication, and real-time monitoring of pharmaceutical items are all made possible by blockchain's decentralized and transparent ledger. Stakeholders at each step in the supply chain may check a product's unique identification to ensure it is genuine and from the right location. Pharmaceutical tracking and supply chain management enabled by blockchain technology aspires to make the pharmaceutical business more trustworthy and secure for patients and other stakeholders by reducing the prevalence of counterfeit pharmaceuticals, increasing transparency, and strengthening compliance.

Security and Privacy in Healthcare Blockchain

In this section, we will explore the key components of security and privacy in healthcare blockchain.

Immutable and tamper-proof data storage

A blockchain designed for the healthcare industry organizes the storage of data in blocks that are cryptographically connected to one another to create a chain. After the information has been stored in a block, it is very difficult, if not impossible, to modify or remove it. The consensus process that is employed in blockchain networks guarantees that all participants agree on the legitimacy of new data before it is added to the chain. This occurs before the new data is added to the chain. Because of this, the integrity and reliability of medical records are improved, and the possibility of unauthorized data alteration or adjustments is decreased.

Encryption and cryptographic techniques

Encryption is a crucial component in ensuring the confidentiality of sensitive data in blockchain-based systems. The use of public key infrastructure, or PKI, is common practice when attempting to set up encrypted communication channels between members of a network. Each participant has a one-of-a-kind set of cryptographic keys (public and private keys), which are put to use for the creation of digital signatures. These signatures guarantee the genuineness of the data and validate the sender's identity. Data that is encrypted and stored on the blockchain is kept secret, and only authorized people in possession of the appropriate keys may access and decode the data.

Access control and permissioned blockchains

Blockchains built for the healthcare industry may take the form of public, private, or permissioned networks. Permissioned blockchains are preferable for use in healthcare applications because they provide for more control over the access granted to data and continue to protect the confidentiality of sensitive information. Within the blockchain network, access control methods have been established to guarantee that only authorized persons or organizations are able to see, add to, or alter the data that is stored there (Al-Sumaidaee et al., 2023).

Privacy-enhancing technologies for healthcare data

Due to the sensitive nature of medical information, protecting patients' privacy is of the highest significance in the healthcare industry. Even inside the confines of a blockchain network, privacy-enhancing technologies (PETs) are used to maintain the confidentiality of patient information (Ismail et al., 2019). The following are some examples of commonly utilized PETs in blockchain applications related to healthcare:

- *Zero-Knowledge Proofs (ZKPs):* ZKPs enable a party to demonstrate the veracity of a claim without disclosing the truth of the claim.
- *Differential Privacy:* To avoid the identification of specific patients while yet allowing for an insightful analysis of the data, this method adds statistical noise to aggregated data.
- *Secure Multi-Party Computation (SMPC):* With the use of SMPC, many people may jointly calculate a function while maintaining the privacy of their individual inputs.
- *Homomorphic Encryption:* With homomorphic encryption, calculations may be performed on encrypted data without having to first decode it.

Challenges and Considerations

The potential of blockchain technology in enhancing security and privacy within the healthcare sector is considerable. However, its widespread adoption is contingent upon addressing various challenges and considering crucial considerations. This section explores the primary obstacles and factors to be considered when implementing blockchain technology in the healthcare industry.

Scalability and performance issues

Blockchain networks, particularly those that are public in nature, encounter inherent constraints in terms of scalability and performance. As the volume of participants and transactions grows, the blockchain may experience a decrease in speed and efficiency. Scalability assumes critical importance in the healthcare sector, given the substantial daily generation of voluminous data (Yaqoob et al., 2021).

Regulatory and legal implications

The healthcare sector is subject to extensive regulations aimed at protecting patient data and promoting ethical conduct. The implementation of blockchain technology necessitates a thorough examination of prevailing regulatory frameworks, data privacy legislation, and compliance obligations. The decentralized nature of blockchain poses challenges in complying with specific data protection regulations, such as the General Data Protection Regulation (GDPR) in Europe and the Health Insurance Portability and Accountability Act (HIPAA) in the United States.

Integration with existing healthcare systems

Healthcare organizations commonly possess established legacy systems that are responsible for the storage and management of patient data. The process of incorporating blockchain technology into these preexisting systems can present challenges in terms of complexity and time requirements. The establishment of interoperability between blockchain and conventional databases is of utmost importance to mitigate the formation of data silos and facilitate smooth data interchange.

Ethical considerations and patient consent

The utilization of blockchain technology for the storage and management of healthcare data gives rise to ethical concerns pertaining to patient consent and data ownership. It is imperative to ensure that patients are adequately educated regarding the manner in which their data will be utilized, the individuals or entities who will possess access to it, and the potential advantages and disadvantages associated with the adoption of blockchain technology (Tandon et al., 2020).

Case Studies and Implementation Examples

This section showcases successful healthcare blockchain initiatives, lessons gained, best practices, and different use cases across healthcare disciplines.

Successful blockchain projects in healthcare

MedRec is an innovative healthcare blockchain technology created by MIT researchers. It improves EHR administration and patient data privacy and interoperability. The initiative addresses fragmented patient data among healthcare providers and a lack of patient control over medical information.

Key Features and Components:

- *Patient-Centric EHRs:*   The MedRec system prioritizes patient-centric electronic health records (EHRs), placing patients at the focal point of their healthcare data. This technology enables patients to exercise full autonomy over their medical records, granting them the ability to selectively disclose designated information solely to authorized healthcare providers.
- *Smart Contracts for Data Access:*   The utilization of smart contracts on the blockchain by MedRec is employed to regulate the authorization and control of patient data. The primary objective is to establish a system that restricts access to specific medical information solely to authorized entities, such as healthcare providers, in accordance with patient consent and predetermined permissions.
- *Patient Consent Management:*   The MedRec system includes a consent management system that allows patients to indicate the individuals or entities authorized to access their medical records and the specific purposes for which such access is granted.

Medical chain is a platform that leverages blockchain technology to facilitate secure telemedicine consultations and the exchange of medical information. The main aim of this project is to tackle the obstacles presented by geographical barriers, with the goal of improving the availability and reach of healthcare services. Furthermore, it aims to prioritize the safeguarding of data privacy and security.

Key Features and Components:

- *Telemedicine Consultations:*   Medical chain facilitates the establishment of secure telemedicine consultations, allowing patients to establish connections with healthcare providers. Patients have the opportunity to engage in conversations regarding their medical conditions, obtain remote diagnosis, and avail themselves of medical guidance from duly licensed professionals.
- *Medical Data Management:*   Medical chain provides a secure platform for patients to store their medical records on the blockchain. This encompasses data such as an individual's medical background, diagnostic findings, prescribed medications, and strategies for treatment.
- *Health Passport:*   Medical chain provides a "Health Passport" functionality that facilitates the consolidation of a patient's medical data, enabling them to

conveniently share their information with healthcare providers, irrespective of geographical constraints.

Lessons learned and best practices

The success of a blockchain project is heavily dependent on the application of lessons learned and best practices as shown in Table 10.2. Teams may improve their ability to overcome obstacles, tighten up security, and boost the overall effectiveness of their blockchain solutions by learning from earlier efforts and putting into practice tried-and-true tactics.

Table 10.2   Lessons learned and their objectives.

Objective	*Key Lessons Learned*
Clearly Define Objectives	Well-defined vision and goals aid in selecting suitable blockchain use cases for healthcare.
Address Real-World Challenges	Successful projects tackle real-world healthcare issues like data security, interoperability, and supply chain streamlining.
Engage Stakeholders Early	Involvement of stakeholders from the beginning ensures the solution meets diverse needs and gains support for adoption.
Privacy and Compliance	Balancing transparency and data privacy while adhering to industry-specific compliance builds trust among users.
Scalability and Performance	Considering scalability and performance from the outset helps handle large volumes of healthcare data.
Integration with Existing Systems	Seamless integration with existing healthcare systems ensures interoperability and reduces workflow disruption.
Education and Training	Providing adequate training to healthcare professionals and users fosters blockchain system acceptance and usability.
Collaboration and Partnerships	Collaboration among stakeholders leads to comprehensive and successful blockchain projects by leveraging expertise and resources.
Proof of Concept and Pilots	Conducting POC and pilot projects provides valuable insights and helps identify potential challenges before full-scale deployment.
Continual Evaluation and Improvement	Regular evaluation of performance, security, and user experience ensures the long-term relevance and effectiveness of the solution.

Conclusion and Future Directions

Blockchain technology has attracted considerable interest in revolutionizing various industries, including healthcare. This chapter explores the potential of blockchain in creating a secure healthcare infrastructure, addressing issues like cyber-attacks and data privacy. Use cases in healthcare, such as data interoperability, patient identity management, electronic health records, and clinical trials, are investigated. Challenges like scalability, legal compliance, system integration, and ethics are discussed. The future of blockchain in healthcare involves incorporating AI and smart contracts for improved efficiency and personalized care. Collaboration among stakeholders is crucial for successful implementation, and blockchain holds great promise in safeguarding healthcare systems and enhancing patient outcomes.

References

Adere E.M. 2022. Blockchain in healthcare and IoT: A systematic literature review. *Array*, 14, 100139.

Al-Sumaidaee G., Alkhudary R., Zilic Z. and Swidan A. 2023. Performance analysis of a private blockchain network built on Hyperledger Fabric for Healthcare. Information Processing and Management, 60(2), 103160.

Chen H.S., Jarrell J.T., Carpenter K.A., Cohen D.S. and Huang X. et al., 2019. Blockchain in healthcare: A patient-centered model. *Biomedical Journal of Scientific and Technical Research*, 20(3), 15017.

Cheng X., Chen F., Xie D., Sun H. and Huang C. et al., 2020. Design of a secure medical data sharing scheme based on blockchain. *Journal of Medical Systems*, 44(2), 52.

Fu J., Wang N. and Cai Y. 2020. Privacy-preserving in healthcare blockchain systems based on lightweight message sharing. *Sensors*, 20(7), 1898.

Gupta A., Bhagat M. and Jain V. 2023. Blockchain-enabled healthcare monitoring system for early Monkeypox detection. *The Journal of Supercomputing*, 1–25.

Ismail L., Materwala H. and Zeadally S. 2019. Lightweight blockchain for healthcare. *IEEE Access*, 7, 149935–149951.

Kumar A., Singh A.K., Ahmad I., Kumar Singh P., Anushree Verma P.K. et al., 2022. A novel decentralized blockchain architecture for the preservation of privacy and data security against cyberattacks in healthcare. *Sensors*, 22(15), 5921.

Lakhan A., Mohammed M.A., Nedoma J., Martinek R., Tiwari P. et al., 2023. DRLBTS: Deep reinforcement learning-aware blockchain-based healthcare system. *Scientific Reports*, 13(1), 4124.

McGhin T., Choo K.K.R., Liu C.Z. and He D. 2019. Blockchain in healthcare applications: Research challenges and opportunities. *Journal of Network and Computer Applications*, 135, 62–75.

Pandey P. and Litoriya R. 2020. Implementing healthcare services on a large scale: Challenges and remedies based on blockchain technology. Health Policy and Technology, 9(1), 69–78.

Pandey P. and Litoriya R. 2020. Securing and authenticating healthcare records through blockchain technology. Cryptologia, 44(4), 341–56.

Pradhan N.R., Singh A.P., Verma S., Kaur N., Roy D.S. et al., 2022. A novel blockchain-based healthcare system design and performance benchmarking on a multi-hosted testbed. *Sensors*, 22(9), 3449.

Prybutok V.R. and Sauser B. 2022. Theoretical and practical applications of blockchain in healthcare information management. *Information and Management*, 59(6), 103649.

Qiu J., Liang X., Shetty S. and Bowden D. 2018. Towards secure and smart healthcare in smart cities using blockchain. In 2018 *IEEE International Smart Cities Conference* (ISC2) (pp. 1–4). IEEE.

Saidi H., Labraoui N., Ari A.A.A., Maglaras L.A. and Emati J.H.M. et al., 2022. DSMAC: Privacy-aware Decentralized Self-Management of Data Access Control based on blockchain for health data. *IEEE Access*, 10, 101011–101028.

Shahnaz A., Qamar U. and Khalid A. 2019. Using blockchain for electronic health records. IEEE Access, 7, 147782–147795.

Tandon A., Dhir A., Islam A.N. and Mäntymäki M. 2020. Blockchain in healthcare: A systematic literature review, synthesizing framework and future research agenda. *Computers in Industry*, 122, 103290.

Villarreal E.R.D., García-Alonso J., Moguel E. and Alegría J.A.H. 2023. Blockchain for healthcare management systems: A survey on interoperability and security. *IEEE Access*, 11, 5629–52.

Xie Y., Zhang J., Wang H., Liu P., Liu S. et al., 2021. Applications of blockchain in the medical field: Narrative review. *Journal of Medical Internet Research*, 23(10), e28613.

Yaqoob I., Salah K., Jayaraman R. and Al-Hammadi Y. 2021. Blockchain for healthcare data management: Opportunities, challenges, and future recommendations. *Neural Computing and Applications*, 1–16.

11

The Future of Healthcare: Data-Driven Trends and Innovation

Wasswa Shafik[1]*

The future of medical care is looked at in this research study with the prism of establishing innovations since any aspect associated with human health and wellness influences individuals to numerous degrees as end users. Starting with a study of exactly how modern technologies can change the health care method is provided ;the research study details these principles. It goes over exactly how IoT gadgets and sensing units can monitor people's crucial indicators, check their problems, and collect wellness details. It likewise takes a look at the function of the Internet of Things (IoT) in medical care. Technologies pertaining to robotics and automation are likewise checked out, stressing on exactly how helpful they could be for clinical treatments, treatment, and senior citizen treatment. The research discovers the opportunities of modern blockchain technology in health care with significantly more information, highlighting its capability to boost information safety, interoperability, and personal privacy. Regulatory, personal information privacy, and honest concerns are covered, attending to the repercussions and troubles of creating innovations in health care moving forward. Finally, for the complete capacity of these modern technologies to be understood, it highlights the demand for continuous research study, cooperation, and hostile regulation.

[1] School of Digital Science, Universiti Brunei Darussalam, Gadong, BE1410, Brunei Darussalam, Dig Connectivity Research Laboratory (DCRLab), Kampala, Uganda

* Corresponding author: wasswashafik@ieee.org

Introduction

The market's quick technical developments have actually caused considerable medical care distribution, monitoring, and experience adjustments over the last few years. These improvements have actually dramatically affected several healthcare-related areas, consisting of personal treatment, medical diagnosis, forecasts, therapy, and information monitoring (Yang et al., 2020). Among one of the most substantial improvements is the advancement of telemedicine. In-person appointments are no longer required because of the improvement of interaction innovation, which allows individuals to talk to clinical experts from another location (Saleemi et al., 2020). Telemedicine has actually made it simpler for individuals to obtain medical care, particularly those living in remote locations or with restricted wheelchairs. It has actually likewise been helpful throughout times of dilemma by allowing people to get clinical recommendations and therapy from the comfort of their homes, for instance, throughout the very early Coronavirus illness (COVID-19) pandemic (Sood et al., 2022).

Enormous quantities of clinical information, consisting of research study write-ups, digital wellness documents (EHRs), and clinical imaging, can currently be checked out utilizing expert system formulas to produce informative details and improve scientific decision-making (Nguyen et al., 2022). AI formulas have actually shown the capacity to anticipate the program of a health problem and are fads and help in creating personalized therapy programs. AI-powered services have actually been confirmed to be exceptionally precise when detecting disorders like skin cancer cells and eye illness, perhaps allowing earlier recognition and far better individual results (Holland et al., 2021).

The IoT has actually had a substantial effect on medical care. IoT tools' smoothen interaction and information exchange capacities, for example, smart clinical tools and sensing units, enhance functional performance in medical care atmospheres. By maximizing procedures and boosting client security, attached gadgets supply real-time tracking, property monitoring, and anticipating upkeep (Richer et al., 2020; Shafik. 2024a). Modern robotic technology has actually progressed medical care, permitting accurate and minimally invasive treatments, helping individual treatment tasks, and sustaining recovery programs. The medical care industry might create and adjust to the altering demands of people and culture by proactively checking out ETs.

Healthcare employees and scientists can progress in clinical development and quicken the development of ground-breaking treatments, medicines, and clinical tools by checking out ETs. Partnerships among doctors, information technology companies, and scientists can advertise multidisciplinary reasoning and ingenious societies in the healthcare ecological community (Shafik. 2024b). Checking out ETs additionally aids the healthcare industry in planning for the future. Healthcare companies might stay in the lead and proactively address transforming individual requirements, market characteristics, and regulative responsibilities by anticipating and accepting brand-new modern technologies (Richer et al., 2020). Figure 11.1 shows healthcare technology.

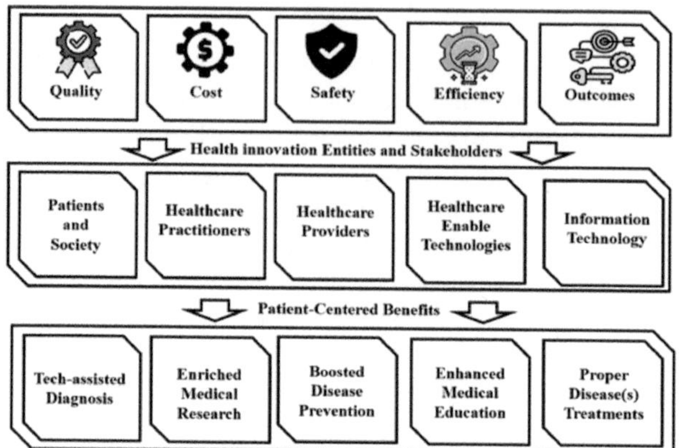

Fig. 11.1   Healthcare innovation

The Chapter Contributions

The chapter presents the following contributions, as summarized below:

- The chapter discusses how IoT devices and sensors can monitor patients, track vital signs, and collect health data highlighting the benefits and challenges of implementing IoT in healthcare, including security and privacy concerns.
- Explores AI applications such as diagnosis and decision support systems, medical imaging analysis, and personalized medicine discussing the applications of augmented and virtual reality in healthcare education, training, and patient care.
- Gives details on the fundamentals of blockchain technology (BT) and its potential applications in healthcare, and discuss how blockchain can enhance data security, interoperability, and patient privacy. Reviews the advancements in genomic sequencing technologies and their impact on personalized medicine and explores the use of genomic data in disease diagnosis, treatment selection, and drug development.
- Explores ETs enabling remote healthcare delivery, such as telemedicine, wearable devices, and mobile health applications, and discuss the benefits of remote healthcare in improving access to care, monitoring chronic conditions, and reducing healthcare costs, and highlight the challenges and considerations in implementing remote healthcare technologies.
- Finally, it discusses the potential future developments and trends in ETs in healthcare and analyzes the challenges and barriers to the widespread adoption of these technologies, including regulatory concerns, data privacy, and ethical considerations.

The Chapter Organization

Section 11.2 presents the Internet of Things (IoT) in healthcare, entailing a definition of the IoT and its relevance in the healthcare sector. Section 11.3 presents artificial intelligence (AI) in healthcare and describes the role of AI in transforming healthcare delivery. Section 11.4 presents robotics and automation in healthcare, examining the use of robotics and automation technologies in various healthcare settings. Section 11.5 presents ETs for remote healthcare, exploring ETs enabling remote healthcare delivery. Section 11.6 illustrates the future implications and challenges and discusses the potential future developments and trends in ETs in healthcare. Finally, Section 1.7 portrays the future impact and challenges.

Internet of Things and Blockchain Technology in Healthcare

Within this section, we present the fundamentals of IoT and BT and their potential applications in healthcare and discuss how blockchain is applied.

BT is a decentralized, open-source structure that makes purchases and information storage space secure and stable. Blockchain is essentially a chain of blocks, each consisting of an encrypted, timestamped document of purchases. A dispersed journal is kept by a network of individuals rather than a solitary entity by attaching these blocks making use of cryptographic hashes (Yang et al., 2020). Health care is among the many markets that this modern technology has the prospective to change.

Blockchain can address crucial information interoperability, safety and security, and personal privacy concerns in the healthcare sector. Handling EHRs is an essential application. Blockchain modern technology can enhance information honesty, protect against unlawful modifications, and help with smooth interoperability between doctors and systems (Saleemi et al., 2020, Shafik. 2023c). Professional tests and studies can additionally make use of blockchain in the healthcare market. Scientists can successfully team up while preserving personal

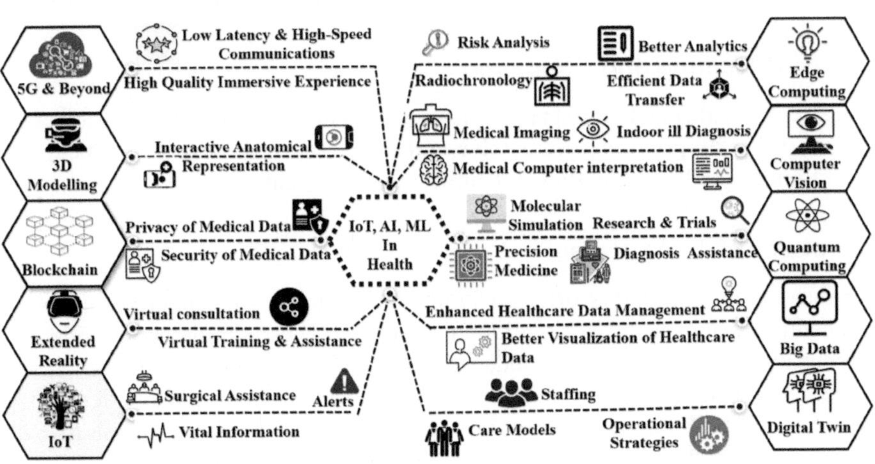

Fig. 11.2   Application of the healthcare enabling technologies in the medical field

privacy information and possession with the help of blockchain, making it feasible to share study information safely and transparently (Sood et al., 2022).

The pharmaceutical field can make use of blockchain to track the whole medication supply chain, guaranteeing the stability and authenticity of drugs. Stakeholders might track a medication's course from manufacturer to supplier to last customer by recording every deal and activity on the blockchain, decreasing the threat of fake medicines, improving personal safety and security, and improving governing conformity (Nguyen et al., 2022). Individuals can safely regulate and share individual health and wellness details via blockchain-based systems, offering medical care experts, scientists, and various other stakeholders accessibility as required (Holland et al., 2021).

Blockchain makes use of some techniques to enhance information safety and security. Initially, since blockchain is decentralized, information is spread among a network of individuals instead of being kept in a solitary database. Decentralized BT disperses information throughout a network of individuals, lowering the opportunity of a solitary factor failing and boosting information safety (Razdan and Sharma. 2022; Shafik. 2023d; Yang et al., 2020). This shields the information's stability and makes it harder for criminals to jeopardize or meddle with it. The blockchain's cryptographic hashing guarantees that each block is attached to the one prior to it, making it hard to alter the information discreetly (Gaobotse et al., 2022). Figure 11.2 demonstrates how wellness allows modern technologies to be utilized in the clinical sector.

Augmented Reality and Virtual Reality in Healthcare

These are quickly progressing modern technologies that can transform different markets, including medical care. They supply immersive and interactive experiences that can boost clinical training, personal treatment, treatment, diagnostics, and more.

Medical Training and Education

Augmented reality and virtual reality innovations change clinical training education and learning by providing immersive and interactive knowing experiences that boost understanding, retention, and ability advancement.

Surgical Skill Development

Virtual reality simulators offer an immersive training atmosphere for surgical procedures that exceeds past traditional strategies. These simulators provide very practical setups; hence, clinical students and cosmetic surgeons can execute intricate treatments securely (Liebeskind. 2023). By replicating the responsive feelings of surgical treatment, haptic responses in modern technology allow individuals to really feel resistance and comments comparable to actual cells. The precise activities, hand-eye control, and spatial understanding needed for effective surgical treatment are created as a result of this experience (Franzén. 2023).

Comprehensive Anatomy Learning

In admiration of these technical devices, pupils can examine these 3D designs of the body from all angles. These complex designs give an interactive technique for learning more about physiological systems, connections, and frameworks. Pupils can essentially modify, check out, and study-specific locations to comprehend complex frameworks that standard books or two-dimensional graphics could not sufficiently depict (Izonin et al., 2023).

Clinical Scenario Simulations

Augmented reality and virtual reality simulations that copy numerous clinical setups offer a risk-free setting for students to exercise their professional abilities and decision-making capabilities. Clinical trainees can exercise diagnosing, creating therapy strategies, and handling people making use of these simulations, which differ from conventional individuals getting in touch with major circumstances (Shafik et al., 2020a). Real-time physical responses and vibrant individual communications are included right into sophisticated simulations to produce an extra sensible discovery atmosphere. To develop self-confidence and capability in real-world professional setups, pupils can attempt different methods, obtain instant comments, and refine their replies (Shafik et al., 2021).

Interprofessional Collaboration Training

Modern virtual reality technologies aid interprofessional education and learning, given that health care is collective. Clinical pupils, registered nurses, pharmacologists, and various other medical care professionals can team up to detect and deal with digital individuals through shared digital scenarios. This communication enhances synergy, understanding of different obligations, and interactions (Hu et al., 2023; Shafik et al., 2020b). Learners participating in multidisciplinary cooperation are much better prepared to take care of intricate clinical situations that need input from various experts.

Soft Skills and Patient Interaction

Past technological efficiency and the advancement of soft abilities essential for patient-centered treatment are assisted by Augmented reality and virtual reality. Clinical pupils can exercise reliable interaction, compassion, and energy, paying attention through online communications with realistic client characters (Hallinan et al., 2023; Ude-Okeleke et al., 2023). They acquire the capability to take care of tough talks, comprehend clients' perspectives, and provide thoughtful therapy. These online experiences offer a protected setup for creating psychological knowledge and a bedside way, eventually increasing patient enjoyment and count (Shopova et al., 2023).

Patient Medical Care

Virtual reality innovation uses immersive experiences that can draw away people's focus from discomfort and pain throughout clinical treatments.

Pain Management

By producing immersive settings that successfully draw people away from discomfort and anxiousness throughout clinical procedures, virtual reality offers a unique means of discomfort administration. People are required to make remarkable online globes making use of the power of virtual reality, which hinders them from thinking of their clinical circumstances and lowers their feeling of suffering (Heydari et al., 2023). By involving people in these exciting experiences, healthcare experts could decrease the requirement for sedatives and pain relievers, possibly improving the whole individual experience and the recovery procedure.

Rehabilitation and Therapy

Personal treatment is reinvented when treatment and rehab programs consist of AR and virtual reality technology. Virtual reality exercises and interactive video games in physical rehabs offer an engaging means for people to be involved even more strongly in their recovery procedure. These satisfying tasks advertise routine adherence to restorative regimens and offer people a stimulating and satisfying electrical outlet for gaining back toughness and movement (Gough et al., 2023). Comparable to this, AR and virtual reality systems give a selection of specialized tasks for cognitive recovery that examine clients' cognitive capabilities in interesting and interactive means, advertising cognitive recovery and healing.

Exposure Therapy

Direct exposure treatment, which deals with fears and anxiety problems, utilizes augmented reality and virtual reality. These modern technologies aid people in ending up being much less conscious of their problems by establishing digital setups that subject clients to their triggers gradually in a secure way (Wang et al., 2023). This approach minimizes phobic responses and boosts individuals' capability to regulate anxiety-provoking occasions by equipping them to face their issues securely.

Patient Education

The natural visualization capabilities of augmented reality and virtual reality offer innovative methods for conveying complex clinical concepts to individuals. With increased facts, physicians might put specific clinical imaging on clients' bodies to provide a physical aesthetic representation of their issues and therapy alternatives (Malik et al., 2023). The interactive technique advertises this joint and educated healthcare trip, enhancing client understanding and decision-making involvement. Individuals can practically exercise complicated surgeries with virtual reality simulations prior to the treatment (Salajegheh et al., 2023). With the help of this thorough sneak peek, individuals can much better understand the surgery, which aids in soothing their worries and enhancing interaction between them and the clinical group.

Mental Health Support

Without effort, imagining difficult clinical principles, AR and VR offer ingenious methods to enlighten clients. Clinical service providers can use thorough clinical imaging of individuals' bodies, making use of increased facts to provide a physical and aesthetic representation of their health problems and therapy choices (Malik et al., 2023). This interactive approach advertises a joint and experienced medical care trip by boosting client understanding and involvement in decision-making. On top of that, virtual reality simulations permit individuals to exercise complicated surgeries ahead of time (Salajegheh et al., 2023). The operation is debunked with an immersive sneak peek, and clients are provided extra expertise, which reduces stress and anxiety and promotes effective conversation between people and physicians.

Diagnostic Imaging

These innovations are transforming analysis imaging by making it possible for interactive and immersive visualization of clinical scans. Clinical employees can utilize enhanced truth to overlay three-dimensional individual check depictions onto their physical atmosphere, supplying a one-of-a-kind sight of complex physiological elements (Hallinan et al., 2023). This assists with medical preparation and boosts understanding of clinical imaging information. Physicians can get three-dimensional scans in virtual reality, permitting an extra all-natural examination of individual composition.

Telemedicine

Augmented reality and virtual reality are changing telemedicine with a brand-new level of interactivity and engagement throughout remote clinical assessments. By graphically stressing essential factors in real-time video clip streams, physicians can utilize increased truth to help people comprehend clinical ideas. Virtual reality advances telemedicine by submerging individuals in electronic depictions of physician seeing or healing experiences (Moulaison-Sandy and Wenzel, 2023). This modern technology enhances client participation by getting rid of geographical restrictions and improving the telemedicine experience by making it a lot more customized and immersive.

Cognitive Rehabilitation

Augmented reality and virtual reality are vital in cognitive rehabs, especially for individuals recovering from mind injuries or cognitive disabilities. These devices give simulations and jobs created to check cognitive capacities, consisting of memory, interest, and analysis (Heydari et al., 2023). AR can supply interactive hints and motivate in an individual's setting that assists with memory recall and work conclusion. On the other hand, virtual reality provides organized and engaging settings for cognitive exercises, boosting the enjoyment and efficiency of treatment. Both techniques sustain practical self-reliance and cognitive recovery.

Pain Distraction and Relaxation

People can place AR or VR tools throughout clinical procedures to move them to serene online landscapes. This immersive diversion substantially reduces the feeling of discomfort and anxiousness, making therapies less complicated to deal with and perhaps removing the demand for sedatives. In addition, virtual reality settings developed for leisure can help individuals take care of persistent discomfort or lower tension (Gough et al., 2023). These innovations use a non-pharmacological technique for discomfort monitoring and psychological wellness by immersing people in calm and immersive settings. Incorporating AR and VR right into these individual treatment setups calls for cautious assimilation, individual education and learning, and recurring assessment (Wang et al., 2023).

Genomics and Precision Medicine

The research of an individual's whole hereditary code, or genome, is referred to as genomics. Discovering details of genetics, variations, and anomalies involves sequencing and assessing Deoxyribonucleic Acid (DNA). Genetics are the plans that identify exactly how our bodies expand, work, and respond to the outdoors. When establishing clinical treatments, accurate medication, or tailored medication, take into consideration a person's special hereditary, ecological, and way of living qualities. Accuracy medication is used to supply personalized treatments that are extra effective and have less damaging impacts rather than taking on a one-size-fits-all technique.

Genomic Sequencing and Cancer Genomics

The core of genomics is genomic sequencing, which entails analyzing an individual's whole hereditary code. It requires identifying the nucleotide series that comprises our DNA. Comprehending hereditary versions and anomalies that influence an individual's health and wellness relies on this comprehensive examination. Cancer cell genomics, utilizing this technique, has actually transformed oncology (Mannell et al., 2023). Medical care specialists create customized medications that match the molecular attributes of growth by thoroughly analyzing the hereditary modifications sustaining cancer cell development. This customized method boosts personal results, diagnoses, and treatment effectiveness.

Bioinformatics and Pharmacogenomics

The large quantity of information generated by genome sequencing calls for much analysis, which is where bioinformatics, a mix of biology and informatics, can be found. Bioinformatics makes use of computational methods and software program devices to amass important understandings from complex hereditary information. Pharmacogenomics is a practical application in which an individual's hereditary account is examined to identify exactly how they reply to medications (Hampel et al., 2023). These details aid physicians in selecting the correct drugs, dos and donts, and treatments, reducing negative effects and enhancing therapeutic outcomes.

Genetic Testing and Rare Disease Diagnosis

Hereditary screening entails taking a look at an individual's DNA for hereditary variants connected with conditions and attributes. It aids in medical diagnosis by disclosing the hereditary reasons for conditions. The medical diagnosis of unusual conditions is an instance (McFarlane et al., 2023). Medical care professionals might offer accurate medical diagnoses, diagnoses and personalized therapy strategies that attend to the underlying root causes of these issues by recognizing the genetic abnormalities that underlie unusual problems.

Genome Editing Tools and Gene Therapy

Genome modifying strategies are changing exactly how people communicate with hereditary products, such as Clustered Frequently Interspaced Brief Palindromic Repeats (CRISPR-Cas9). These strategies make it feasible to customize certain genetics, which provides excellent possibilities for fixing hereditary imperfections and healing illness from the inside out. Genetic treatment is important in placing restorative genetics right into a person's cells to take care of congenital diseases (Subbiah. 2023).

Predictive and Preventive Medicine and Nutrigenomics

Genomics sustains anticipating and preventative medication by establishing a person's hereditary sensitivity to particular conditions. This info makes it possible for very early treatments, way-of-life adjustments, and personalized safety nets. Nutrigenomics is an interesting application that checks out exactly how hereditary variants impact responses to diet plans and nourishment (Xiong et al., 2023). By understanding these connections, tailored nutritional guidance can be developed, enhancing wellness results based on an individual's hereditary tendencies.

Prenatal and Neonatal Genomics and Infectious Disease Genomics

Genomic evaluation of unborn children and neonates is a prenatal and neonatal genomics element. Because of this, hereditary dangers can be determined, assisting in the routing of treatments and providing an understanding of possible wellness trajectories from the earliest phases of life. On the other hand, transmittable condition genomics checks out the genes of the virus (Hampel et al., 2023; Xiong et al., 2023). Scientists find out vital details that can help them develop specialized drugs, vaccinations, and approaches to eliminate transmittable conditions by checking out the hereditary selection and advancement of these conditions.

Enabling Technology for Remote Healthcare

Numerous innovations that allow the shipment of clinical solutions, appointments, and support from a range are needed to allow remote health care.

Telemedicine Platforms

Telemedicine systems are full systems that permit remote interaction between people and doctors. Physicians and people can seek advice in real-time utilizing these systems' protected video clip conferencing solutions. They, in addition, use features like visit organizing, document sharing for medical records, and encrypted messaging for asynchronous discussion (Liebeskind. 2023). Systems for telemedicine make it possible for Medical Insurance Mobility and Liability Act-certified interactions to get over geographical obstacles and offer a range of clinical therapies from another location.

Mobile Health (mHealth) Apps

mHealth applications are mobile programs produced to help with numerous aspects of health care. These applications can check a person's key indicators, medicine program, and signs and symptoms. They use educational sources and devices to help individuals take care of persistent illnesses like diabetes mellitus or high blood pressure. Some mobile health and wellness applications likewise allow online appointments, enabling clients to get in touch with healthcare experts from any area (Hallinan et al., 2023).

Remote Patient Monitoring Devices

Remote Person Tracking (RPM) tools collect and quickly send client wellness details to clinical personnel. These gizmos might consist of glucometers, high blood pressure displays, and wearable sensing units, to name a few. Individuals with persistent conditions, those recouping from surgical treatment, and those in jeopardy of health and wellness occasions can all be kept an eye on from another location by RPM (Ude-Okeleke et al., 2023). If an individual's important indications differ from the common arrays, healthcare experts can obtain alerts, making it possible for timely treatments and aggressive treatment administration.

Virtual Reality and Augmented Reality

Countless opportunities exist in which virtual reality and AR innovations enhance remote medical care. Comprehensive direction for physician and healing client experiences can be given through virtual reality simulations of clinical atmospheres. Physicians can envision clinical information throughout online assessments and make it possible for remote partnerships for medical preparation thanks to AR, which lays over electronic details in the real setting (Heydari et al., 2023). These modern technologies, individual communications, and clinical education and learning enhance the precision of remote medical diagnosis.

Internet of Things Sensors

IoT sensing units are incorporated right into home devices, wearables, and clinical gadgets. They develop a networked ecological community that collects details on individuals' physical and psychological health. These sensing units can track medicine conformity place drops, control home environments (for instance, temperature level for older people), and offer details regarding clients' everyday tasks (Piano et al., 2023; Shafik. 2023b). When abnormalities are discovered, this information can increase signals and educate doctors regarding their people's wellness.

Wearable Health Devices

Health and wellness criteria can be constantly kept an eye on with wearable innovation, such as smartwatches, health and fitness trackers, and clinical wearables (instances are displayed in Figure 11.3). They keep an eye on different points, consisting of heart rate, exercise, and rest behaviors. By motivating significantly healthier routines and helping individuals recognize their wellness patterns, these tools sustain clients' general health (Heydari et al., 2023; Shafik 2023a). Furthermore, they provide handy details that could assist physicians in choosing therapy choices and treatment methods.

Remote Diagnostics

Utilizing remote analysis devices like tele-ultrasound and tele-radiology, clinical employees can translate clinical pictures from another location. Radiologists, for example, can assess Armed Forces Recruiting Info Collection, CT checks, or X-rays from another location and use quick monitoring (Eggmann et al., 2023). These devices give fast diagnostics in remote or underserved areas where accessibility to professional clinical competence might be restricted.

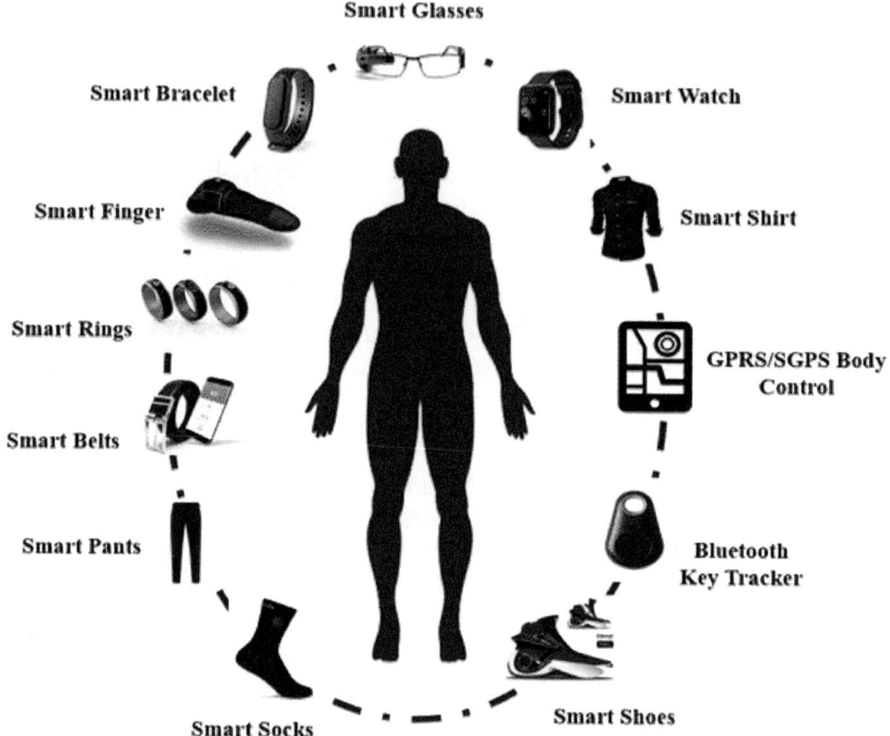

Fig. 11.3 Sampled wearable medical electronics

Electronic Health Records Systems

Online EHR systems keep clinical information regarding people, offering medical care specialists safe accessibility to extensive documents. In order to preserve the connection of treatment, remote doctors can examine individuals' medical records, examination searching, and therapy strategies (Gardner, 2023). The simplicity of accessibility to EHR systems promotes decision-making and interaction between people and healthcare experts.

Future Implications and Challenges

Customized health care is becoming the standard thanks to the merging of genes and accurate medication. Therapy strategies will certainly be made especially for each individual's hereditary account, enhancing performance and decreasing negative effects.

Future Implications

Personalized Treatment Paradigm

The way in which clinical therapies are provided will transform because of genomics and the accuracy of medication. Medical care will certainly highlight tailored therapy programs dealing with an individual's hereditary make-up, way of living, and ecological conditions as opposed to a one-size-fits-all technique (Piano et al., 2023). This standard change intends to lower negative effects while boosting healing efficiency. Take into consideration the opportunity that customizing medication based on hereditary pens that influence medication metabolic rate might lead to even more exact and reliable therapies (Malik et al., 2023).

Disease Prevention and Early Detection

Future advancements in genes can substantially change methods of disease discovery and avoidance at an early stage. Medical care experts can use preventative treatments and lifestyle adjustments that reduce the possibility of disease advancement by taking a look at a person's hereditary tendency to have certain problems (Eggmann et al., 2023). Additionally, genetic screening makes early ailment discovery feasible prior to signs and symptoms showing up.

Advancements in Drug Development

The area of medication advancement will undergo a transformation thanks to genomic explorations. Scientists can discover certain hereditary targets and paths for healing treatments by comprehending the hereditary structure of conditions (Gardner, 2023). These details perhaps improve the medicine advancement procedure and increase the success price of medical tests, increasing the advancement of customized drugs that target the underlying root causes of illness.

Genomic Data-Driven Research

Genomic data sources are widely prepared to sustain ground-breaking research study tasks. Scientists can find links between genetics, ailments, and therapy results by assessing hereditary information from numerous populations (Jayaraman et al., 2023). These explorations might lead the way for finding fresh restorative targets and producing accurate medication approaches for numerous conditions, including complex and uncommon conditions.

Improved Public Health Strategies

Genomic info at the populace degree can substantially modify public health plans. Healthcare authorities can adjust inoculation programs to certain hereditary vulnerabilities by reviewing hereditary variants throughout various teams, raising the performance of booster shot initiatives (Guilherme et al., 2023). Furthermore, populace genomics' searches can aid public health programs far better in addressing typical congenital diseases.

Challenges of Data-driven Trends and Innovation

Data Privacy and Security

Making sure solid information, personal privacy, and protection are important issues is critical since genomic information consists of delicate and exclusive information. The comprehensive collection and circulation of hereditary information elevates problems pertaining to unlawful access gain to information violations and the abuse of this information for differentiating or business goals (Ruiz and Velásquez 2023). Cutting-edge file encryption innovations, rigorous regulations, and extra understanding of information safety treatments will certainly be required to strike an equilibrium between information sharing for research study functions and shielding individuals's privacy.

Data Interpretation Complexity

Academics and medical care specialists find it challenging to understand hereditary information due to its intricacy. Advanced bioinformatics strategies, computational sources, and hereditary understanding are called for to evaluate massive quantities of hereditary information to produce substantial understandings (Sanchez-Pinto et al., 2023). Offering exact and scientifically appropriate analyses of hereditary information will certainly be essential to stopping wrong medical diagnoses or therapy suggestions.

Health Disparities

Reasonable accessibility to advanced innovations and treatments will certainly be a huge trouble for genomics in the future. Wellness injustices might aggravate if detailed populaces cannot get hereditary screening, accurate medications, and treatments due to monetary, geographical, or social restraints (Hulsen et al., 2023). Wellness differences need to be attended to by plans that sustain accessibility to genomics for all social teams, framework growth, education and learning.

Regulatory Frameworks

Producing ideal regulative structures to supervise genomes and accurate medication presents a major problem. It is essential to stabilize and cultivate development, assure individual safety and security, and promote moral standards (Cussat-Blanc et al., 2023). Regulatory authorities should adapt to the regularly transforming genomics landscape for hereditary screening, information exchange, scientific tests, and the recommendation of customized medications.

Psychosocial Impact and Ethical Considerations

The psychological effect of genomics ends up being significantly tough to deal with as it offers possibly life-altering truths. For individuals and family members, hereditary screening outcomes might create stress and anxiety, unpredictability, or emotional suffering (Cussat-Blanc et al., 2023). To allow individuals to make a decision concerning hereditary screening carefully and to handle the ramifications of the details they discover, it is necessary to supply correct psychosocial assistance, genetic counseling, education and learning. Partnerships between scientists, healthcare experts, policymakers, ethicists, client supporters, and modern technology designers will certainly be essential to get rid of these challenges (Xiong et al., 2023).

Future Research Directions, Lessons Learnt, and Conclusion

ETs are essential for determining the future of the healthcare sector, which is undergoing an ongoing change. The following are the top eight trends for ETs in healthcare in the future:

Future Research Directions

AI and ML have actually changed the healthcare market by evaluating huge quantities of clinical information, progressive diagnostics, projecting illness results, helping in therapy preparation, and boosting client surveillance. Healthcare experts can take advantage of utilizing AI-powered formulas to help them make even more exact and educated judgments, enhancing client results (Vukmirovi et al., 2018). The Internet of Medical Things, the network of sensing units and clinical devices, is called the IoMT. It allows real-time event tracking, and evaluation of individual wellness specifications. IoMT devices can boost persistent disease administration, preventive therapy, and remote person tracking, as displayed in Figure 11.4.

Lessons Learnt from the Chapter

The impact of ETs on healthcare is highlighted in the following lessons, along with the necessity of carefully navigating the opportunities and difficulties that come with their implementation, as summarized.

- ETs have actually transformed medical care like IoT and AI, boosting medical diagnosis, therapy preparation, and individual tracking. These innovations enhance individual results by allowing healthcare employees to make even more enlightened and exact choices.
- High-performance computers and huge information analytics have actually accelerated the procedure of locating brand-new medicines and conducting clinical research studies. The capacity to analyze large quantities of clinical information, making use of high-performance computers and progressed analytics, has actually accelerated clinical research study and the advancement of brand-new therapies.

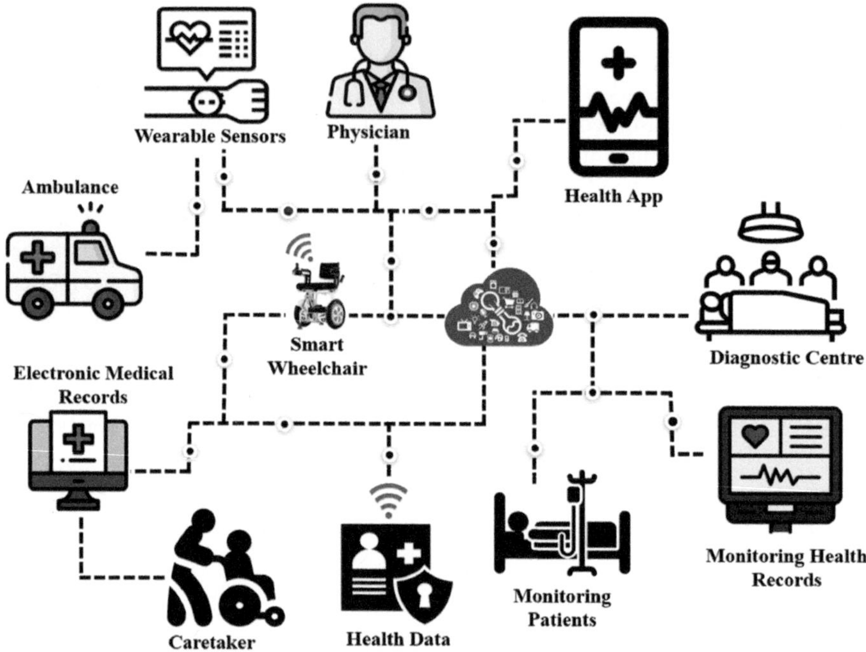

Fig. 11.4 Real-time artificial intelligence of the internet of medical things ecosystem implementation

- Customized medication has actually transformed therapy techniques thanks to genomic and various other omics information. The development of modern omics technologies and various other facets of genes have actually opened brand-new opportunities for individualized medication.

- Mobile phones and wearables, like mHealth applications and wearables, have actually equipped people to handle their health and wellness. These innovations advertise precautionary treatment and individual involvement by making it possible for individuals to check their health and fitness degrees, take care of persistent conditions, and access health-related info.

- People can currently handle their wellness utilizing mobile phones and wearables like mHealth software applications. With the help of these modern technologies, individuals might check their health and fitness degrees, care for persistent conditions, and get health-related details that advertise preventative treatment and individual engagement.

- Information safety and security, personal privacy, regulative conformity, and equivalent accessibility to modern technology are very important factors to consider. As healthcare executes ETs, it is crucial to focus on information security and protection, adhere to lawful needs, and ensure equivalent accessibility to innovation.

Conclusion

The quick development of ETs has actually reinvented the healthcare market and considerably boosted individual treatment and outcomes. Lessons from the effects of these innovations underscore their transformative capacity and the need to take certain facets into account. Targeted and individualized medication is ending up being advanced thanks to high-performance computers and huge information analytics. Wearable modern technologies and mobile phone applications allow people to boost their health and wellness, while digital health and wellness documents and interoperable systems improve treatment control and client security. Nonetheless, it is critical to concentrate on lawful conformity, personal information privacy and protection, and equivalent accessibility to modern technology. Health care experts need to proceed with their training education and learning to manipulate the capacity of ETs correctly. Exploring ETs and investing cash in RandD will certainly aid medical care services to remain at the leading edge of development while improving client treatment and providing a one-upmanship. While dealing with issues in these locations, BT can improve person personal privacy, interoperability, and information safety. Nevertheless, for ETs to be extensively utilized in medical care, scalability, policy, and criteria should be addressed.

References

Cussat-Blanc S., Castets-Renard C. and Monsarrat P. 2023. Doctors in Medical Data Sciences: A New Curriculum. *International Journal of Environmental Research and Public Health*, 20(1). https://doi.org/10.3390/ijerph20010675.

Eggmann F., Weiger R., Zitzmann N.U. and Blatz M.B. 2023. Implications of large language models such as ChatGPT for dental medicine. In *Journal of Esthetic and Restorative Dentistry*. https://doi.org/10.1111/jerd.13046.

Franzén A. 2023. Big data, big problems: Why scientists should refrain from using Google Trends. Acta Sociologica (United Kingdom). https://doi.org/10.1177/00016993221151118.

Gaobotse G., Mbunge E., Batani J. and Muchemwa B. 2022. Non-invasive smart implants in healthcare: Redefining healthcare services delivery through sensors and emerging digital health technologies. *Sensors International*, 3. https://doi.org/10.1016/j.sintl.2022.100156.

Gardner J. 2023. Imaginaries of the data-driven hospital in a time of crisis. *Sociology of Health and Illness*, 45(4). https://doi.org/10.1111/1467-9566.13592.

Gough P., Bown O., Campbell C.R., Poronnik P. and Ross P.M. et al., 2023. Student responses to creative coding in biomedical science education. Biochemistry and Molecular Biology Education, 51(1). https://doi.org/10.1002/bmb.21692.

Guilherme A.A., de Lara Machado W., Monteiro Sanchez G. and de Oliveira Rosa L. 2023. The development and initial validation of an instrument measuring levels of violence suffered and practiced by students in higher education. Policy Futures in Education, 21(2). https://doi.org/10.1177/14782103221097208.

Hallinan C.M., Habibabadi S.K., Conway M. and Ann Bonomo Y. 2023. Social media discourse and internet search queries on cannabis as a medicine: A systematic scoping review. *PLoS ONE*, 18(1 January). https://doi.org/10.1371/journal.pone.0269143.

Hampel H., Gao P., Cummings J., Toschi N., Thompson P.M. et al., 2023. The foundation and architecture of precision medicine in neurology and psychiatry. In Trends in Neurosciences 46(3). https://doi.org/10.1016/j.tins.2022.12.004.

Heydari F., Nobakht M., Vahedian-Azimi A., Mirzamani S.S., Moradian S.T. et al., 2023. Developing the marine medicine syllabus for medical sciences students: a multiphase design study. BMC Medical Education, 23(1). https://doi.org/10.1186/s12909-023-04461-4.

Holland J., Kingston L., McCarthy C., Armstrong E., O'dwyer P. et al., 2021. Service robots in the healthcare sector. In Robotics (Vol. 10, Issue 1). https://doi.org/10.3390/robotics10010047.

Hu F., Wen J., Zheng D. and Wang W. 2023. Travel medicine in hospitality: an interdisciplinary perspective. *International Journal of Contemporary Hospitality Management.* https://doi.org/10.1108/IJCHM-05-2022-0574.

Hulsen T., Friedecký D., Renz H., Melis E., Vermeersch P. et al., 2023. From big data to better patient outcomes. In *Clinical Chemistry and Laboratory Medicine,* 61(4). https://doi.org/10.1515/cclm-2022-1096.

Izonin I., Kutucu H. and Singh K.K. 2023. Smart systems and data-driven services in healthcare. In *Computers in Biology and Medicine,* 158. https://doi.org/10.1016/j.compbiomed.2022.106074.

Jayaraman P., Crouse A., Nadkarni G. and Might M. 2023. A Primer in Precision Nephrology: Optimizing Outcomes in Kidney Health and Disease through Data-Driven Medicine. In *Kidney360,* 4(4). https://doi.org/10.34067/KID.0000000000000089.

Liebeskind D.S. 2023. Editorial: Rising stars in precision medicine 2021: imprecise medicine is unethical in the big data era. In *Frontiers in Medicine,* 10. https://doi.org/10.3389/fmed.2023.1181788.

Malik S., Muhammad K. and Waheed Y. 2023. Nanotechnology: A Revolution in Modern Industry. In *Molecules,* 28(2). https://doi.org/10.3390/molecules28020661.

Mannell K., Fordyce R. and Jethani S. 2023. Oaths and the ethics of automated data: limits to porting the Hippocratic oath from medicine to data science. *Cultural Studies,* 37(1). https://doi.org/10.1080/09502386.2022.2042577.

McFarlane R., Galvin M., Heverin M., Mac Domhnaill É., Murray D. et al., 2023. PRECISION ALS— an integrated pan European patient data platform for ALS. *Amyotrophic Lateral Sclerosis and Frontotemporal Degeneration.* https://doi.org/10.1080/21678421.2023.2215838.

Moulaison-Sandy H. and Wenzel A.G. 2023. The Records Data Ecosystem in Humanities and Human Sciences Scholarship. *Portal,* 23(1). https://doi.org/10.1353/pla.2023.0000.

Nguyen D.C., Pham Q.V., Pathirana P.N., Ding M., Seneviratne A., Lin Z., Dobre O. and Hwang W.J. 2022. Federated Learning for Smart Healthcare: A Survey. ACM Computing Surveys, 55(3). https://doi.org/10.1145/3501296

Piano M., Diemer K., Hall M., Hui F., Kefalianos E. et al., 2023. A rapid review of challenges and opportunities related to diversity and inclusion as experienced by early and mid-career academics in the medicine, dentistry and health sciences fields. *BMC Medical Education,* 23(1). https://doi.org/10.1186/s12909-023-04252-x.

Razdan S. and Sharma S. 2022. Internet of Medical Things (IoMT): Overview, ETs, and Case Studies. In IETE Technical Review (Institution of Electronics and Telecommunication Engineers, India) (Vol. 39, Issue 4). https://doi.org/10.1080/02564602.2021.1927863.

Ruiz R.B. and Velásquez J.D. 2023. Artificial intelligence at the service of the health of the future. *Revista Medica Clinica Las Condes,* 34(1). https://doi.org/10.1016/j.rmclc.2022.12.001.

Salajegheh M., Hekmat S.N. and Malekpour-Afshar R. 2023. Identification of alternative topics to diversify medicine, dentistry, and pharmacy student theses: a mixed method study. *BMC Medical Education,* 23(1). https://doi.org/10.1186/s12909-023-04031-8.

Saleemi M., Anjum M. and Rehman M. 2020. Ubiquitous healthcare: a systematic mapping study. *Journal of Ambient Intelligence and Humanized Computing.* https://doi.org/10.1007/s12652-020-02513-x.

Sanchez-Pinto L.N., Bhavani S.V., Atreya M.R. and Sinha P. 2023. Leveraging Data Science and Novel Technologies to Develop and Implement Precision Medicine Strategies in Critical Care. In *Critical Care Clinics.* https://doi.org/10.1016/j.ccc.2023.03.002.

Shafik W. 2023a. A Comprehensive Cybersecurity Framework for Present and Future Global Information Technology Organizations. In *Effective Cybersecurity Operations for Enterprise-Wide Systems* (pp. 56-79). IGI Global. https://doi.org/10.4018/978-1-6684-9018-1.ch002.

Shafik W. 2023b. Cyber security perspectives in public spaces: Drone case study. In *Handbook of Research on Cybersecurity Risk in Contemporary Business Systems*. https://doi.org/10.4018/978-1-6684-7207-1.ch004.

Shafik W. 2023c. Making Cities Smarter: IoT and SDN Applications, Challenges, and Future Trends. *In Handbook of Research on Opportunities and Challenges of Industrial IoT in 5G and 6G Networks*. https://doi.org/10.4018/978-1-7998-9266-3.ch004.

Shafik W. 2023d. Artificial Intelligence and Blockchain technology enabling cybersecurity in telehealth systems. *Artificial Intelligence and Blockchain Technology in Modern Telehealth Systems*, 285-326. IET. https://doi.org/10.1049/PBHE061E.

Shafik W. 2024a. Introduction to ChatGPT. Advanced Applications of Generative AI and Natural *Language Processing Models* (pp. 1-25). IGI Global. https://doi.org/10.4018/979-8-3693-0502-7.ch001.

Shafik W. 2024b. Navigating Emerging Challenges in Robotics and Artificial Intelligence in Africa. *Examining the Rapid Advance of Digital Technology in Africa* (pp. 124-44). IGI Global https://doi.org/10.4018/978-1-6684-9962-7.ch007.

Shafik W., Matinkhah S.M. and Ghasemzadeh M. 2020a. Theoretical Understanding of Deep Learning in UAV Biomedical Engineering Technologies Analysis. *SN Computer Science*, 1(6). https://doi.org/10.1007/s42979-020-00323-8.

Shafik W., Mojtaba Matinkhah S., Etemadinejad P. and Sanda M.N. 2020b. Reinforcement learning rebirth, techniques, challenges, and resolutions. *International Journal on Informatics Visualization*, 4(3). https://doi.org/10.30630/joiv.4.3.376.

Shafik W., Mojtaba Matinkhah S., Shokoor F. and Nur Sanda M. 2021. Internet of things-based energy efficiency optimization model in fog smart cities. *International Journal on Informatics Visualization*, 5(2). https://doi.org/10.30630/joiv.5.2.373.

Shopova D., Yaneva A., Bakova D., Mihaylova A., Kasnakova P. et al., 2023. (Bio)printing in Personalized Medicine—Opportunities and Potential Benefits. In *Bioengineering* (Vol. 10, Issue 3). https://doi.org/10.3390/bioengineering10030287.

Sood S.K., Rawat K.S. and Kumar D. 2022. A visual review of Artificial intelligence and Industry 4.0 in healthcare. *Computers and Electrical Engineering*, 101. https://doi.org/10.1016/j.compeleceng.2022.107948.

Subbiah V. 2023. The next generation of evidence-based medicine. *Nature Medicine*, 29(1). https://doi.org/10.1038/s41591-022-02160-z.

Ude-Okeleke R.C., Aslanpour Z., Dhillon S. and Umaru N. 2023. Medicines Related Problems (MRPs) Originating in Primary Care Settings in Older Adults – A Systematic Review. In *Journal of Pharmacy Practice* (Vol. 36, Issue 2). https://doi.org/10.1177/08971900211023638.

Vukmirović A., Rajnai Z., Radojičić M., Vukmirović J. and Milenković M.J. et al., 2018. Infrastructural model for the healthcare system based on ETs. *Acta Polytechnica Hungarica*, 15(2). https://doi.org/10.12700/APH.15.1.2018.2.2.

Wang R.S., Maron B.A. and Loscalzo J. 2023. Multiomics Network Medicine Approaches to Precision Medicine and Therapeutics in Cardiovascular Diseases. *Arteriosclerosis, Thrombosis, and Vascular Biology*, 43(4). https://doi.org/10.1161/Atvbaha.122.318731.

Xiong X., Lv G., Jiang B. and Lu K. 2023. Editorial: From randomized clinical trials to real-world data and big data sciences: Generating evidence-based medicine for value in western and herbal medicines. In *Frontiers in Public Health* (Vol. 11). https://doi.org/10.3389/fpubh.2023.1129399.

Yang G., Pang Z., Jamal Deen M., Dong M., Zhang Y.T. et al., 2020. Homecare Robotic Systems for Healthcare 4.0: Visions and Enabling Technologies. *IEEE Journal of Biomedical and Health Informatics*, 24(9). https://doi.org/10.1109/JBHI.2020.2990529.

Index